Maria Treben

Health through God's Pharmacy

Advice and experiences
with medicinal herbs

PUBLISHER WILHELM ENNSTHALER, STEYR (AUSTRIA)

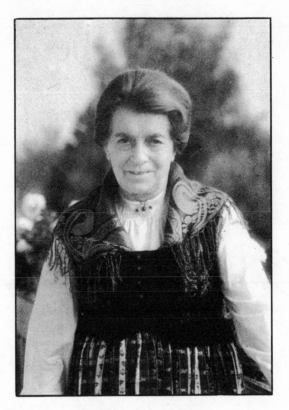

MARIA TREBEN

The information contained herein is not presented with the intention of diagnosing or prescribing, but is offered only as information for use in maintaining and promoting health in cooperation with a physician. In the event that the information presented in this book is used without a physician's approval, the individual will be diagnosing for himself. No responsibility is assumed by the author, publisher or distributors of this publication for use of the information contained herein in lieu of a doctor's services. No guarantees of any kind are made for the performance or effectiveness of the preparations mentioned in this publication.

Cover design, colour plates and drawings by Robert SCHOELLER, Vienna
Translated from the German

24th Edition 1994

ISBN 3 85068 124 6

Preface

At a time, when the majority of mankind has moved away from life's natural ways, when illness, caused by a changed attitude to life, threatens, we should turn again to medicinal herbs which God in His Greatness has provided for us since time immemorial. The Abbé (Father) Kneipp in his books says: **"There is a plant for every illness!"** Everyone is able to improve his or her health by the timely gathering and use of herbs, be it as a tea drunk daily or as a course of treatment, using the extracts as a friction or a compress, as an addition to baths, as a poultice and so on. Once the decision to use herbs is taken, it is wise to start with herbs which purify the blood, such as Chicory, Dandelion, Ramsons, Speedwell and Stinging Nettle. Such treatments are never harmful, when the herbs are used exactly as prescribed. If they bring only slight or no relief and help, it might be possible that field disturbances exist in the home or workplace. In this case an experienced diviner should be consulted, to find the areas which are free of disturbances.

At the first signs of discomfort, fever and other clear symptoms of an illness, it is essential to **consult a doctor immediately for diagnosis and advice**. It is also essential to have the course of a serious illness and the healing process controlled conscientiously by a doctor.

The modern medicine is slowly starting to turn to the field of natural healing emerged at the 25th International Congress for Continuing Education of the German Federal Chamber of Doctors and the Austrian Chamber of Doctors in March, 1980, in Badgastein, Austria, in which approx. 1500 doctors participated.

Dr. Carl **Alken**, professor at the University of Saarland, West Germany, explains modern medicine's increasing awareness of the curative properties of nature as follows: "After World War II, doctors were virtually powerless, for example, in cases of tuberculosis and renal failure. Then came the big change with the **introduction of antibiotics** – and today we have to deal with the negative consequences of the partly excessive and wrong use of this '**Blessing**'. To this is added the immense increase in fungus diseases caused by too much medication and by other environmental influences which upset the normal biological balance."

For years I have been following medical conferences and conventions, the conclusions of which are also covered in newspapers. **Many responsible doctors warn of the overuse of pills.** Time and again it is pointed out, how dangerous **pain killers** can become. Many people take them without medical supervision and this sometimes causes serious damage to organs. For example, medication for lowering the blood pressure, taken for a long period of time, is conducive to breast cancer, as established by three research teams, working independently of each other in Boston, Bristol and Helsinki.

I would like to tell you about the **effects and medicinal properties of plants** and share with you my experiences of the last few years since this book was first published in Austria and Germany, and give you a helping hand on your way to health. To find a way out of the hopelessness of ill health by one's own strength and free will is, thanks to nature's medicinal herbs, humanly elevating. To win back one's health, and to bear responsibility for oneself, elevates human dignity to such a degree that the sick person is taken halfway to recovery from the **hopelessness of his sick life**.

Time and again I have been asked how I acquired the knowlegde and use of herbs. I cannot give a precise answer. As a child I spent my school holidays with the family of a forest ranger, where I experienced, well beyond my age, the interrelationships of nature. I was able to distinguish the different plants and knew their names, but then the significance of medicinal plants was unknown to me. My mother, an enthusiastic Kneipp follower, strove to let us children grow up in a natural way.

When I was a young girl two experiences impressed themselves on my mind. A 40 year old widow, mother of three children, had **leukaemia (leukemia)** and was discharged from hospital as incurable with about three days to live. Her sister, anxious about her, went to see a herbalist, taking a sample of the sick woman's urine. The herbalist said, quite startled: "Only now you bring me this morbid water!" – the herbs she gave, to be used by the sick woman, helped. A medical examination 10 days later showed no sign of leukaemia.

Another similar case occurred at the same time. A 38 year old woman, mother of four children, suffered from leukaemia and hers was a hopeless case too. She, too, used the appropriate herbs. Every day she prepared a tea and kept it in several jugs. Whenever she passed a jug, she took a sip, thinking: if it does not help, it does no harm either. The medical examination 10 days later showed no **sign of leukaemia**!

These examples show how important it is to **drink large amounts of herb tea every day, when suffering from a seemingly incurable illness**. From then on I was certain that **medicinal herbs can bring relief even for serious diseases**.

In 1961 my dear mother died and since then I have the distinct feeling of being **pushed into herbalism**. Gradually I acquired knowledge and experience. It was as if I was guided by a higher power. The Virgin Mary, especially, helper of the sick, was showing me the way. My trust in Her, prayers said before an old wonderful painting of Her, which I acquired in a strange way, have always helped, when I was in doubt.

So I endeavour to not only show you the herbs and their medicinal properties, but above all the omnipotence of a Creator in whose hands we exist. In sickness, we look for His help and comfort and use the humble herbs He has provided; it is He who guides us, so we may live according to His will.

I would like to emphasize finally that I have tried hard in every respect to present all my experiences for man's utilization. I have a favour to ask: **Do not ring me, write to me or come to see me!** The precise index in this book will put you on the **way to using the right herbs**.

Another thing: **I do not sell herbs** and therefore do not take orders. Herb farms, special chemists and health food stores provide them.

Grieskirchen, May 1980

MARIA TREBEN

Temperature	C.	F.	Linear Measures		
Boiling point	100°	212°	1 millimetre (mm.)	≅	0.04 inch
	90°	194°	1 centimetre (cm.)	≅	0.4 inch
	80°	176°	1 metre (m.)	≅	39.4 inches
	70°	158°	1 inch (in.)	≅	25.4 millimetres
	60°	140°	1 foot (ft.)	≅	30.5 centimetres
	50°	122°	1 yard (yd.)	≅	0.9 metres
	40°	104°			
	30°	86°	**Weights**		
	20°	68°	1 gramme (gm.)	≅	15.4 grains
	10°	50°	1 kilogramme (kg.)	≅	2.2 pounds
Freezing point	0°	32°	¼ pound (lb.)	≅	120 grammes
			1 ounce (oz.)	≅	30 grammes

Liquids

1 litre (l.) ≅ 1.8 pints   1 pint (pt.) ≅ 0.6 litres

CONTENTS

GENERAL INFORMATION

The right way to gather, store and prepare herbs

GATHERING

A knowledge of herbs is essential for gathering. Gathering should be undertaken at the right time, at the right place and in the right manner.

Experience shows that best results are obtained with freshly picked herbs, which are absolutely essential for success with serious illnesses. Fresh herbs can be picked in early spring, sometimes from the end of February till into November. Some are even found during winter under the snow (e.g. Greater Celandine), if one knows where to look.

For winter a not too large supply of dried herbs is stored. For this purpose they are gathered at the time of their greatest vigour.

For **FLOWERS** this is the beginning of flowering.
For **LEAVES** before and during the time of flowering.
ROOTS are dug out in early spring or autumn.
FRUITS are gathered at the time of ripening.

At the same time observe the following hints: Pick only healthy, clean plants free from pests. Gather herbs on sunny days in dry condition, when the dew has evaporated.

Fields and meadows treated with chemical fertilizer, the banks of dirty, contaminated waters, railway embankments and the neighbourhood of heavy traffic roads and motorways (highways) and of industrial plants, are no places for gathering.

Treat Nature with consideration! (Don't pull plants out by their roots, don't make a mess.) Some plants are protected by law. There are enough herbs with the same effectiveness which are not protected (e.g. Auricula – Cowslip).

Do not crush flowers and leaves while gathering and do not use plastic bags and containers. The herbs begin to sweat and later become black during drying.

DRYING

The herbs are not washed before drying. They are spread thinly on cloths or unprinted paper and dried as quickly as possible in the shade or in warm, ventilated rooms (attics). Roots, barks or very fleshy parts of plants are often dried in a warm oven. The oven temperature should not exceed 35° C. = 95° F. It is best to cut roots which are well washed (Mistletoe and Willow-herb are also cut) before drying.

Only fully dried herbs – they crackle and break when bent – can be stored for winter. For storage, glass jars or sealable cartons are the most appropriate. Plastic and metal containers are to be avoided. The herbs should be protected from light (use coloured glass jars, green being the most appropriate).

Keep a supply for **one** winter only. With time the herbs lose their healing power. Every year presents us with a new harvest of herbs.

Methods of Preparation

HERB TEAS

Infusions: Fresh herbs are cut and the prescribed quantity placed in a teapot or other non-metallic container. Water is brought to the boil and poured over the prepared herbs. Fresh herbs are steeped for a very short time only (half a minute will suffice). The tea has to be quite light; light yellow or light green. Dried herbs are steeped somewhat longer (one to two minutes). A tea prepared in this manner is substantially more wholesome and also more pleasing to the eye.

Roots are placed in the required amount of cold water, brought to the boil and steeped for 3 minutes.

The daily requirement of tea is poured into a thermos flask and the prescribed quantity sipped during the day. In general one takes one heaped teaspoon of herbs in one quarter litre of water (= 1 cup), or otherwise as prescribed for the individual plants.

Cold Infusions: Some herbs (e.g. Mallow, Mistletoe or Calamus) should not have boiling water poured over them, as their healing power is lost through the influence of heat. A tea from these herbs is obtained by cold infusion. The prescribed quantity of the respective plants is steeped in cold water eight to twelve hours (mostly overnight), then warmed (to drinking temperature only) and the daily requirement kept in a thermos flask, rinsed beforehand with hot water. A cold infusion mixed with a hot infusion provides a means of extracting the most of value from medicinal plants. The herbs are steeped overnight with half of the prescribed amount of water and strained in the morning. The other half of the prescribed amount of water is brought to the boil, poured over the herb residue and strained again. Cold and hot infusions are now mixed. The active substances which are soluble either only in cold or only in hot water are obtained in this way.

TINCTURES (ESSENCES)

Tinctures are also extracts, which are won with 38% to 40% strength corn or fruit spirits. A bottle or other sealable container is loosely filled with the appropriate herbs and rye whisky or wodka poured over them. Leave standing well sealed in a warm place (ca. 20° C. = 68° F.) for fourteen days or longer, shake frequently, then strain and squeeze out the residue. Tinctures are taken internally as drops diluted with herb tea or applied externally as compresses or massages.

FRESH JUICES

Fresh juices of herbs are suitable for taking internally in drop form or for dabbing on affected parts of the body. They are made fresh daily. Poured into small bottles and well sealed, they will keep for a few months, however, if stored in the refrigerator.

PLANT PULP

Stems and leaves are crushed to a pulp on a wooden board with a wooden rolling pin. Spread on a piece of linen, place on the affected part of the body, bind with a cloth and keep warm. This poultice can remain on overnight.

HERB POULTICES

In a pot bring water to the boil, hang over it a sieve in which are laid fresh or dried herbs, and cover. After some time, take the softened, warm herbs, put them on a lightly woven cloth and place on the affected part. Everything is covered with a woollen cloth and bound fast with further cloths. No feelings of cold should arise. Very effective are warm Horsetail poultices. Warm poultices are left on for two hours or overnight.

OINTMENTS AND OILS

Two heaped double handfuls of herbs are finely chopped. 500 gm. of lard are heated as if for frying schnitzel. The herbs are stirred into this hot fat, allowed to crackle briefly, stirred around, the pan is removed from the hotplate, covered and cooled overnight. The next day the whole is warmed lightly, filtered through a linen cloth and the still warm ointment poured into previously prepared glass jars or ointment pots.

Oils are prepared as follows: Flowers or herbs are loosely placed in a bottle up to the neck, cold-pressed olive oil is poured over them till the oil stands two finger widths above the flowers or herbs. Let stand 14 days in the sun or near a stove.

HERB BATHS

Full Bath: The appropriate herbs are steeped overnight in cold water. One bucketful (6 to 8 litres) of fresh herbs or 200 gm. of dried herbs is needed for a bath. This is heated and strained the next morning and poured into the bath water. Soak in it for 20 minutes. The heart must be above the water. After the bath do not dry off but wrap yourself in a bath towel or robe, go to bed and lie there for one hour perspiring.

Sitz Bath: For a sitz bath take only half a bucketful of fresh herbs or approx. 100 gm. of dried herbs and proceed as for a full bath. The bath water must cover the kidney region. Observe the instructions for the particular herbs.

The water from the full bath as well from the sitz bath can be re-warmed and used twice more.

SWEDISH BITTERS COMPRESS

A piece of cottonwool or gauze, of a size compatible with the affected area, is dampened with drops of **Swedish Bitters** and laid on the affected area, which has been well covered with lard or Calendula ointment to prevent the alcohol drying out the skin. Over this a somewhat larger piece of plastic may be placed to protect the clothing, then a warm cloth or a bandage is tied over the whole. The compress is left to take effect for two to four hours, depending on the illness and tolerance. If the patient can tolerate it, the compress can remain on overnight. After removal of the compress the skin is powdered. Should sensitive people develop skin irritations the compress must be applied for a shorter period or discontinued for a while. People who are allergic to plastic may dispense with it and only use the cloths. In no case should one forget to grease the skin before applying the compress. Should itching occur, use Calendula ointment.

With these compresses it is not necessary to lie in bed, for, if the area is well bandaged, one can sit or move about the house.

Abbé	= Father	haemorrhoid	= hemorrhoid
anaemia	= anemia	homoeopathic	= homeopathic
diarrhoea	= diarrhea	leucorrhoea	= leucorrhea
gynaecologist	= gynecologist	leukaemia	= leukemia
haematoma	= hematoma	oedema	= edema
haemophilia	= hemophilia	oesophagus	= esophagus
haemorrhage	= hemorrhage	seborrhoea	= seborrhea

MEDICINAL HERBS FROM GOD'S PHARMACY

AGRIMONY (Agrimonia eupatoria)

Common names: Sticklewort, Cockle Burr, Church Steeples.

It grows in sunny dry places, on hedgebanks, on sides of fields, woods and paths, on wastelands and near ruins. Its small yellow flowers cluster on slender spikes, similar to the Mullein. The whole plant is covered with soft hair, the leaves near the ground are often 10 cm. long and pinnate. Agrimony, which can reach a height of 80 cm., belongs to the same family of plants as Lady's Mantle. The plant is gathered when in flower, from June to August. The history of this herb, as with many others, goes back a long way and it was known to the Ancient Egyptians.

Agrimony has great healing properties for **inflammation of the throat and mouth**. Remember this in cases of **tonsillitis, throat disorders, thrush or inflammation of the mucous membrane of the mouth**. Gargling with this tea clears the voice for singers and public speakers.

The leaves are excellent for **anaemia and wounds** and are used successfully for **rheumatism, lumbago, digestive trouble, hardening of the liver and spleen disorders**. Drink up to 2 cupfuls a day.

Everyone should make the effort to have an Agrimony bath once or twice a year (see "directions"). Children with **scrofulous sores** should have one daily.

Agrimony, because of its astringent and healing qualities, is one of our most valued herbs. Dr. Shierbaum says: "A cup of Agrimony tea drunk three times a day is a remedy for **enlargement of the heart, stomach and lungs as well as kidney and bladder** disorders, if you drink it over a period." Agrimony ointment, which is used in a similar way to Calendula ointment, is of benefit in **varicose veins and sores on the lower legs** (see "directions").

For **disorders of the liver** mix 100 gm. of Agrimony, 100 gm. of Bedstraw and 100 gm. of Woodruff (Asperula odorata). Drink a cup of this tea on an empty stomach and sip 2 cupfuls during the day.

DIRECTIONS

Infusion: 1 teaspoon of Agrimony to ¼ litre of boiling water, allow to draw for a short while.

Herb Bath: 200 gm. of herbs for 1 bath (see General Information "bath").

Infusion for liver disorders: Blend equal parts of Agrimony, Bedstraw and Woodruff. Use 1 heaped teaspoon to 1 cup of water, infuse for a short time.

Ointment: 1 heaped double handful of finely chopped leaves, flowers and stems to 250 gm. of lard (see "ointments" in General Information).

BEDSTRAW (Galium)

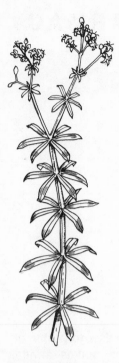

Common names: Clivers, Goosegrass, Yellow Bedstraw, Maid's Hair, Cheese Rennet, Hedge Bedstraw and Lady's Bedstraw.

There are several species: **Galium aparine**, commonly known as Clivers or Goosegrass, grows in meadows, fields and hedges and reaches a height of 60 to 160 cm. Its leaves are placed in whorls and the flowers are greenish white. The stem is covered with little hooked bristles by which it fastens itself to nearby plants.

Galium verum, the True Bedstraw called also Yellow Bedstraw, Maid's Hair, Cheese Rennet, grows in some parts in higher altitudes and in other parts on dry banks, chiefly near the sea. It has small bright yellow flowers on upright stems and grows to a height of 60 cm. This plant exudes a strong honey-like odour and is best gathered in July.

Galium mollugo, Hedge Bedstraw, has dainty yellow white flowers with a faint honey-like odour. It is found on banks and near paths and is mostly prostrate at the time of flowering.

I want to emphasize again that fresh herbs have a greater medicinal value. Even in winter the fresh shoots of Galium mollugo are found under the dry grass in snow-free places.

All three species have similar medicinal qualities and are used the same way.

Bedstraw tea rids the **liver, kidney, pancreas and spleen** of toxic wastes. When suffering from a disorder of the **lymphatic system**, one should drink this tea daily. It is also beneficial for **anaemia, dropsy and stitch in the side**. Used externally this tea is of benefit in many **skin disorders, wounds, boils and blackheads**. It makes an excellent wash for the face as it **tightens the skin**. The freshly pressed juice of Bedstraw, brushed on the affected parts of the skin and left to dry, is very beneficial.

In popular medicine Bedstraw is recommended for **epilepsy, hysteria, St. Vitus dance, nervous complaints, surpressed urine, gravel** and stones. For **goitre**, gargling with this tea throughout the day is effective. A woman told me she had not only lost the goitre, but her **thyroid gland** is now also working normally.

Every year I meet my friends, a couple from Vienna, at a "Kneipp" spa. When we got together in 1979, I found that the woman had a rather noticeable **goitre**. She was afraid of an operation. I recommended Bedstraw. This is infused and, still warm, is deeply gargled as often as possible daily. In February 1980 we met again at the "Kneipp" spa and behold, the goitre was no longer there. Overjoyed she told me that her husband had repeatedly collected fresh Bedstraw for her. From the beginning she perceived that the goitre became gradually smaller until it disappeared completely.

In recent times, cases of **constriction of the vocal chord** have increased. It appears these cases are caused by a virus. Gargling and rinsing with Bedstraw tea brings swift relief. According to the Swiss Abbé Kuenzle, it is also a reliable remedy for serious **kidney disorders**, even if other remedies have failed — especially if Bedstraw is mixed in equal proportions with Golden Rod and Yellow Dead Nettle. In this case the effect shows very quickly. He talks of 14 days. The tea is infused, and half a cup is taken on an empty stomach 30 minutes before breakfast, then the rest is sipped throughout the day. For serious disorders 4 cups a day are taken.

In old times, Bedstraw was very much esteemed by women for **disorders of the uterus**. To ease childbirth, it was laid in the bed in their difficult hours. As the story goes, this was later attributed to the Virgin Mary. As "Our Lady's Bedstraw", She placed it in Her bed. From another legend, She placed it as a soft pillow in Jesus' crib. A Silesian legend tells that She took it, as it was not eaten by the donkey. There is truth in this. Although cows like to eat it, pigs and donkeys won't touch it.

The Abbé Kuenzle tells in his writings of a 45 year old man who suffered from a serious **kidney disorder** which worsened. Finally one kidney had to be removed, the other one was also affected and did not function normally. The man then began a treatment with Bedstraw tea. Daily he drank 4 cups of the previously mentioned tea mixture of Bedstraw, Golden Rod and Yellow Dead Nettle. Frequently he sipped his tea, whereupon his complaint completely cleared up. This same tea mixture is used for all **kidney disorders**.

While the noted botanist, Richard Willfort, in his book "Health through Medicinal Herbs" points out that rinsing with and drinking Bedstraw tea is an excellent remedy for **cancer of the tongue**, just as the freshly pressed juice mixed with butter is a remedy for cancerous growth and **cancer-like skin disorders**, Dr. Heinrich Neuthaler writes in "The Herb Book" the following about Bedstraw: "The white flowering Bedstraw is recommended for cancer in some districts even today — a nonsense that cannot be opposed strongly enough."

For your judgement on this matter, I would like to place before you, esteemed reader, a few experiences with Bedstraw. About 10 years ago I learned of a dentist who suffered from **cancer of the tongue**. After the operation he lost a lot of weight and was to have had X-ray therapy in Vienna. I recommended gargling with Bedstraw tea. A week later I learned that the therapy was no longer necessary and that he recovered more and more from the illness. In a short time he was well.

Somewhat later I heard from a 20 year old woman who also suffered from **cancer of the tongue**. She was advised to consult a doctor in Carinthia (Austria). He promised her that she would get well within 5 years and gave her a herb tea which she showed me one day. I recognized it as Bedstraw. To save her the expense of going to Carinthia, I showed her the Bedstraw growing wild, so that she could gather it herself. She recovered from this terrible illness.

Still another example: It was at the end of March when a young woman from Vienna told me that her mother, 63 years old, was very ill and was to have a second operation on April 19. Six months before, a **cancer-like tumour** suddenly grew in her larynx. The doctor had hidden the truth from her, telling her it was a goitre and thus she had her first operation. For six months everything went well. But then she experienced terrible pain in her left arm which continued day and night. Her hand was swollen, arm and hand were without feeling so that she could not even hold a piece of paper. To ease her pain, the doctor who performed the first operation advised a second operation on April 19, as previously mentioned, in which he intended to cut the nerves between the neck and the collar bone to at least free her from the worst of the pain. He said that medically there was no other help. Despite that, I recommended that the woman drink Bedstraw tea and gargle with it. Besides, I recommended a tea mixture of 300 gm. Calendula, 100 gm. Yarrow and 100 gm. Stinging Nettle (1½ litre per day, every 20 minutes 1 sip) and also rubbing with Bedstraw ointment. You can imagine my happy surprise when I learned that the pain had subsided after 4 days. Up to April 19, the woman had regained feeling in her arm and hand and was able to move both. The doctor was astounded when the daughter asked him not to perform the second operation. He was visibly impressed when she gave him an accurate account of the herb treatment. He said: "Your mother should continue with it." After a time, I was told the woman was doing very well and looking after her family of six.

By treating **cancer-like growths** healing is possible. In recent times there has been an increase in malignant **skin disorders** that show as dark, sharply outlined rough marks. Presumably it is a question of infection. In this case treatment with fresh juice of Bedstraw and Calendula ointment is successful. Without doubt, a blood cleansing tea of Calendula, Stinging Nettle and Yarrow should be used with it.

A woman from Upper Austria had a small **lump** on the floor of the palate and terrible pain in the whole area of the mouth. Through rinsing with Bedstraw tea, the lump disappeared after four days and with it the pain.

The assertion that the use of Bedstraw for such illnesses is nonsense cannot be justified. Certainly it is not the herbs alone that bring help; it is God Almighty who assists in it. Finally everything lies in God's hands!

DIRECTIONS

Infusion:	¼ litre of boiling water is poured over 1 heaped teaspoon of Bedstraw, infused for a short time.
Fresh Juice:	Fresh Bedstraw is washed and, still wet, put into the juice extractor.
Ointment:	Sufficient fresh juice is stirred into butter (room temperature) to provide an ointment-like consistency. Store in refrigerator.

BUTTERBUR, UMBRELLA PLANT (Petasites officinalis)

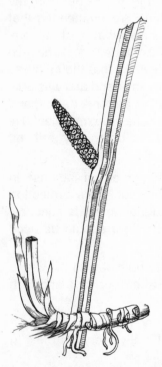

Common names: Bog Rhubarb, Flapperdock. – Butterbur grows on the edges of rivers and woods, in ditches and marshy meadows. It is much larger than the Coltsfoot, which belongs to the same family. The leaves grow to hat size, are slightly scalloped and covered with grey down on the underside. The dirty-white to pale pink flowers, shaped like little baskets, sit densely on the upper part of the stems.

The fever reducing roots, which had gained a great reputation during the time of the plague, are gathered before the time of flowering. The tea promotes perspiration and is used for **fever, shortness of breath, gout and epilepsy**. 1 to 2 cups are sipped during the day.

The large, fresh leaves are applied not only for **sprains, dislocations and sore feet**, but also for every kind of **burn, malignant ulcer and wound**.

DIRECTIONS

Infusion: One level teaspoon of roots is soaked in cold water overnight, warmed and strained in the morning.

Applications: Fresh, washed leaves are crushed and applied. This is repeated several times a day.

CALAMUS, SWEET FLAG (Acorus calamus)

Common names: Sweet Sedge, Sweet Rush, Sweet Root, Myrtle Grass, Sweet Myrtle.

This aquatic plant grows by ponds, lakes, marshes and the banks of quiet waters. The rhizomes out of which numerous swordshaped leaves shoot up to 1 metre high, creep horizontally through the mud at water's edge. The flat scape carries in its middle a cone-shaped, greenish to brownish yellow spadix. The root, the thickness of a thumb and up to 1 metre long, has a pungent, bitter taste when fresh. When dried the taste is milder. The roots are gathered in early spring or late autumn.

Calamus roots are not only used, because of their strenghtening effects, for **overall weakness of the digestive system and flatulence as well as colic**, but are also helpful for **glandular disorders and gout**. The roots **stimulate a sluggish stomach and intestine and dissipate excess mucus**. As well one can recommend them for **slow metabolism and underactivity of the intestine, anaemia and dropsy**.

Extremely thin people, who have lost weight but not through lack of good food, should drink Calamus root tea and occasionally take a Calamus root full bath. Calamus **improves the appetite,** helps in **kidney disorders** and is a good remedy for **cleansing the whole system**. The tea even helps children who suffer from **indigestibility of grain**, which occurs more and more in recent times. The dried roots, chewed slowly, help **smokers to break the habit. Weak eyes** are strengthened if the freshly pressed juice of the Calamus roots is brushed over the closed eyelids from time to time, the juice being left on the lids for a few minutes and rinsed off with cold water.

Repeatedly I have been able to help in cases of **chilblains** and other forms of **frostbite**, with warm Calamus baths. The roots are steeped overnight in cold water and next day brought to the boil. Infuse for five minutes. Then bathe the affected part for 20 minutes in the somewhat cooled (not too hot) infusion. It can be warmed and re-used up to four times. These baths also help those who suffer from **cold hands and feet,** but in these cases the infusion is used as hot as possible.

A 36 year old man could not regain his strength after a tumour on the liver had been removed. In intervals of 4 to 5 weeks, he had attacks of high fever, due to **tubercles in the intestines**. His deeply troubled mother-in-law told me of his hopeless illness. Here, too, Calamus has helped. It is understandable that in such serious cases the tea has to be drunk for weeks, if not for months.

On a mountain hike I met a couple, who, laden with heavy backpacks, were walking uphill. They wanted to spend a few relaxing days in a non-serviced hut. On a rest spot I joined them and I learned the following:

A year ago the man, 1.85 metre tall, in his late fifties, had become a skeleton, without knowing the reason of his illness. Weighing only 45 kilo, he, in company of a nurse, stepped into the surgery of his doctor, who was telephoning another doctor, and heard: "I am sending you my most hopeless patient – **cancer of the lungs**." So, unwittingly, this man learned the diagnosis of his illness. Afterwards someone advised him to chew Calamus roots to break his smoking habit and to drink Yarrow tea, mornings and evenings. Slowly his weight increased and since he felt better, he did not return to the doctor. About half a year later he again went to the surgery of his doctor; who was most taken aback, since he had thought this man dead. "What did you do?" was all he could say. "Chewed Calamus roots and drank Yarrow tea", replied the man. "Calamus roots?, where do you find them?" "They are sold in herbal shops for a few shillings."

The man at this time had reached his normal weight of 86 kilos and it was half a year later that he undertook a mountain hike, carrying a fully laden backpack, when I met him.

Every time I think of his story, mentioning it in my talks or noting it down, as for you now, it seems to me a Godly Providence and I am touched to my innermost. My mother was very ill, she had indescribable pains in the intestines and the doctor told me one day, I should expect the worst – **cancer**. This was at a time I had little to do with herbs, although even then I used natural remedies and never took pills. The doctor's words troubled me deeply. I was hardly able to accomplish the usual work. Against my habit – my day begins at 6 o'clock in the morning and ends at about 11 o'clock at night – I retired to bed shortly after 8 p.m. As I was thinking about the hopeless state of my mother, the door opened, my husband came in, put a small radio at my bedside and said: "So that you are not alone." Shortly afterwards a voice on the radio said: "This is your family doctor speaking. With Calamus roots every **disorder of the stomach and the intestines** is cleared up, be it **stubborn, old or malignant**. Take a level teaspoon of Calamus roots and soak them overnight in a cup of cold water. Warm the liquid slightly in the morning, strain and take one sip of it before and one sip after each meal. That makes 6 sips a day, more should not be taken. The tea should be warmed in a waterbath before each use. This remedy refers to the entire **gastro-intestinal tract, including liver, gallbladder, spleen and pancreas**." Overjoyed, I related this to my mother the next morning, but she said with a resigned movement of the hand: "No one and nothing can help me." I got the Calamus roots and used them as described above. It borders on a miracle, when I tell you that already after 14 days all discomfort had subsided. Weekly my mother now gained 400 gm. She had lost a lot of weight before. Because of this occurrence I gradually became interested in herbalism and was able to help in many hopeless cases. Particularly the Calamus roots brought about startling results again and again.

Where there is too much or too little **acid in the stomach**, the Calamus roots even it out.

A woman from Vorarlberg, the western part of Austria, suffered from **stomach pains** for 2 years and could not be without pills. Following my advice, she took 6 sips of Calamus root tea a day and after 3 days the pain was gone; it has not recurred.

Another woman from Lower Austria, suffered from **duodenal ulcers** for years. To be able to cope with the pain, she relied very much on pills. She could not tolerate solid foods and had no appetite. Told about Calamus roots, she took the recommended 6 sips daily. The pain steadily subsided and, after 5 weeks, had gone completely, her appetite returned and she could join the other members of her family in a hearty meal.

An elderly priest suffering from **diarrhoea** for years, had resigned himself to the situation. Following my advice he began to take 6 sips of Calamus root tea daily. In a short time he was back to normal.

A small boy, who, despite a strict diet, suffered from **diarrhoea (diarrhea)** got well after taking 6 sips of Calamus root tea, his appetite returned and he gained a few pounds. His mother was overjoyed.

A man suffering from **bloody diarrhoea** for 10 years had turned, understandably, from a happy carefree person into a miserable one. Everything he had tried all these years was without success. He was pensioned off still fairly young. Before Easter he started, at first suspiciously, to take 6 sips of Calamus root tea daily and besides this he drank 2 cups of Calendula tea. My surprise was great when I received a letter from his wife telling me he had started work again at the beginning of June.

DIRECTIONS

Infusion: The Calamus root tea is only prepared as a cold-infusion. A level teaspoon of Calamus roots is soaked in ¼ litre of cold water overnight, lightly warmed in the morning and strained. Before using, warm the tea in a waterbath.

Fresh juice: Fresh roots are cleaned thoroughly and, still wet, put in a juice extractor.

Full bath: About 200 gm. of Calamus roots are soaked in 5 litres of cold water overnight, brought to the boil the next day, allowed to infuse and added to the bath water (see General Information "full bath").

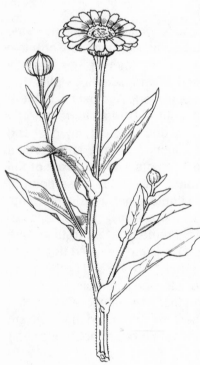

CALENDULA, MARIGOLD (Calendula officinalis)

Common names: Pot Marigold, Mary Gowles, Golds.

Calendula has a noteworthy place among our native herbs. It belongs to the plants which are beneficial in cancer and cancerlike growths. It is found in many gardens in the country, sometimes growing wild on wastelands. Since its healing powers have become recognized again and are in demand, it is now met not only in gardens, but also in fields. Calendula reaches a height of 30 to 40 cm. Its flowerheads are bright yellow to orange. Stems and leaves are fleshy and sticky to the touch. There are several varieties with full flowerheads, with dark or light stamens. The medicinal value is the same. Should its flowerheads be closed after 7 o'clock in the morning, it will rain the same day. It was considered a rain indicator in earlier times.

In folk medicine the plant's flowers, stems and leaves are gathered and used. Gathering should occur in bright sunshine, when its healing powers are at their best. It can be picked fresh in the garden well into late autumn, if free from mildew.

Calendula strongly resembles our Arnica but is superior in its healing power. Arnica should only be used under medical supervision, since the tea could do more harm than good to people with heart trouble. On the other hand, Calendula tea can be drunk without worry. As a **blood cleanser**, it is a great helper in **infectious hepatitis**. 1 to 2 cups a day work wonders. Calendula **cleanses, stimulates circulation** and improves the healing of **wounds**.

A man accidentally put his hand in a circular saw. He had great **pain in the wounds**, after release from the hospital. I heard about it and told him to use Calendula ointment. He was enthusiastic about the results and told me that the pain, which had cost him many sleepless nights, had disappeared after a short time. His wife now plants Calendula in the garden every year.

On a visit, the lady of the house showed me her legs covered with **varicose veins**. I fetched Calendula from her garden and prepared the ointment. The residue I put immediately on her legs (the residues can be used 4 to 5 times). She spread the ointment, the thickness of the back of a knife, on a piece of linen and bandaged her legs with it. You will be surprised, when I tell you that, 4 weeks later, when she visited me at home, the varicose veins had disappeared. Both legs had nice smooth skin. A nun told me that she saw a woman in the street with especially bad varicose veins and advised her to use Calendula ointment. Great was her surprise when, after a month, the same woman joyfully showed her her legs, smooth and free of varicose veins.

The ointment brings swift relief in **phlebitis, varicose ulcers, fistulas, frost bites and burns**. Use the ointment and also the residue of ointment preparations for **ulcers on the breast**, even if they are malignant.

An aquaintance of mine had to have her breast removed. While she was in hospital, I prepared Calendula ointment. Later she used it on her huge **wound from the operation**, whereby the great tension of the wound was quickly eliminated. In a check-up her **scars** from the operation, compared to the scars of other patients, showed such a beautiful heal that she needed only part of the prescribed ray treatment.

The Calendula ointment is also excellent for **Athlete's foot**. Many letters I have received bear this out, especially in cases where all other remedies were of no avail. A decoction of the fresh herb can also be used with success. Should **fungus infestation** start around the area of the genitals, bathe the affected area or use sitz baths. Take 50 gm. dried or 2 heaped double handfuls of fresh Calendula per sitz bath.

A woman from Stuttgart wrote that her husband had suffered from **Athlete's foot** and what had they not tried . . . baths, ointments, powders, none showed results. Then he tried Calendula ointment. After 8 days the open parts had healed and stayed that way. Besides the ointment, a Calendula tincture (see "directions") should be prepared. This tincture diluted with boiled water is especially suited as a compress for **wounds, contusions, bruises and sprains, even for festering or cancer-like sores, bedsores, ulcers and swellings**.

Not only does the Abbé Kneipp believe in Calendula as a natural remedy for malignant growth, but also well known physicians like Dr. Stäger, Dr. Bohn, Dr. Halenser and others. Dr. Bohn names the Calendula as the most important remedy in **cancer illnesses** if it is too late for an operation and recommends the daily drinking of Calendula tea for a prolonged period. The freshly pressed juice of Calendula can be used successfully even in **cancer of the skin. Strawberry marks**, covered with the fresh juice several times a day for a prolonged period, can be made to disappear; the same goes for **pigment spots and brown spots** on elderly people, also rough, **cancerlike skin patches**.

In recent times the American physician and scientist Dr. Drwey points out the unique healing quality of Calendula in **cancer**; he was able to note good success with Calendula.

Internally, Calendula as a tea, is used for **gastro-intestinal disorders, stomach cramps and stomach ulcers, as well as inflammation of the large intestine, dropsy and blood in the urine**. It is excellent for **virus infections** and bacteria in the urine.

What wonderful results the use of the tea of fresh Calendula has is noted in a letter a physician sent to me: "A small 2½ year old girl became very sick after repeated polio inoculations. She had chronic diarrhorea, loss of weight, visual weakness and difficulties with food. In a clinical checkup, **paratyphoid fever** was diagnosed and the child was therefore under clinical supervision. One week after drinking tea, made of fresh Calendula flowers and some homoeopathic medicines, the child was substantially better. The examination for typhoid bacillus, carried out three times shortly afterwards, was negative for the first time."

Since Calendula is also beneficial for **infectious hepatitis**, it is an excellent remedy in **disorders of the liver**. Flowers, leaves and stems are brewed with boiling water. The tea should not be sweetened. For the above mentioned disorders drink 3 to 4 cups a day, about a tablespoonful every quarter of an hour. A tea made from 1 tablespoon of flowers to ¼ litre of water will **expel worms**. The juice of the fresh stem gets rid of **warts and scabies**, the boiled infusion heals **herpes and glandular swellings**, if the affected parts are bathed in it. The tea, drunk regularly **purifies the blood**. The eyes, bathed with an eye bath of the lukewarm tea, are strengthened.

Cancerlike ulcers and growths, cracked feet, ulcerated legs, thigh ulcers and also malignant, suppurating, non-healing **wounds** are helped by washing with an infusion of equal parts of Calendula and Horsetail. Use a heaped tablespoon of this blend to ½ litre of water.

To stress the unique effect of Calendula tea I would like to cite a few more successes. A nurse who suffered from **inflammation of the large intestine** for eight years, had an appointment with a specialist. She was advised to take the Calendula tea as per my book. For 4 days she sipped 2 cups of Calendula tea during the day. She could hardly believe it when after this short use of Calendula all the complaints were gone.

A nun told me she suffered from **diarrhoea**. Although she drank Camomile tea, it did not get better. Only after she had used Calendula tea was there an improvement.

A nun in Bavaria suffered from **Athlete's foot** for 15 years and also repeatedly from **phlebitis**. Through the application of Calendula ointment she experienced finally a healing of her feet.

Scabs in the nose can be easily remedied with Calendula ointment. Note: Should there be an aversion to lard, good vegetable fat may be used. A bit of cooking oil is added to the still warm mass, to make the ointment smoother.

DIRECTIONS

Infusion: 1 heaped teaspoon of herbs to ¼ litre of water.

Sitz bath: Two heaped double handfuls of fresh or 100 gm. of dried herbs for one sitz bath (see General Information "sitz bath").

Washings: 1 heaped tablespoon of herbs to ½ litre of water.

Tincture: 1 handful of flowers are macerated in 1 litre of alcohol. Keep in the sun or at about 20° C. = 68° F. for 14 days.

Ointment: 2 heaped double handfuls of Calendula (leaves, stems, flowers) are finely chopped. 500 gm. of lard are heated and the chopped Calendula is added, stirred, the pan removed from the stove, covered and left to stand for a day. The next day it is warmed, filtered through a piece of linen and poured into previously prepared clean jars.

Fresh juice: Leaves, stems and flowers are washed and, still wet, put into the juice extractor.

CAMOMILE (Matricaria chamomilla)

Common names: German Camomile, Wild Camomile, True Camomile, Scented Mayweed.

It grows on clay soils, arable land, hillsides, in glades, clover-, potato-, corn-, and wheatfields. After snow rich winters and wet springs, it is found in abundance. Because of the increased use of chemical fertilizers and herbicides, our valuable Camomile is more and more eradicated. The hollow receptacle at the base of the blossom distinguishes it from the Roman Camomile. The scent is aromatic and pleasant. A closer description of this well-known plant is undoubtedly unnecessary. Gather the flowerheads from May to August, preferably in the bright noon sun. It is no exaggeration if I cite the Camomile as a "cure-all" especially for babies. In any case, the child should be given Camomile tea if it suffers from **cramps and stomach aches.** The tea is of help in **flatulence, diarrhoea, eruptions, stomach troubles and gastritis, in menstrual disorders, cessation of menstrual flow and in all abdominal disorders, insomnia, inflammation of the testicles, fever, wounds and toothache.**

Camomile produces **perspiration, is soothing and antispasmodic.** It is antiseptic and anti-inflammatory, especially in cases of inflammation of the mucous membranes. Externally Camomile is used as a compress and a wash for **inflamed eyes, conjunctivitis, moist and itching skin eruptions, wounds,** and as a **gargle for toothache.** Anyone who starts feeling aggravated should drink a cup of Camomile tea and soon the wonderfully soothing and sedative effect is felt. Very much recommended is a warm Camomile pillow applied to aching parts.

Camomile baths and washings are most beneficial to the whole **nervous system.** After severe illnesses or for states of exhaustion, its soothing and quieting effect is soon felt. Even as a beauty aid Camomile has its merit. The face washed with a decoction of Camomile once a week will soon show a healthier and softer glow. A decoction used as a **hair conditioner,** especially on blond hair, will make it manageable and give it a beautiful shine.

Camomile helps the movement of the bowels without purging and is therefore indirectly beneficial for **haemorrhoids** to which Camomile ointment can be applied externally. This ointment may also be used to promote the healing of wounds. **Colds and maxillary sinusitis** are soon better if Camomile steam is inhaled. After such a treatment one must understandably remain warm.

The ancient Egyptians dedicated the Camomile to the Sun-God because of its fever-reducing effect and the oil of Camomile was used as a rub for **neuralgia and rheumatic pains** – the name Matricaria comes from the latin "mater" = mother – and, as the name implies, was used for female disorders. In old herbals one reads that the oil of Camomile takes away the **tiredness of limbs** and the boiled flowers, applied to an **ill bladder**, ease the pain.

The Swiss Abbé and herbalist Kuenzle tells of a village woman known as "Camomile Witch" to whom people came in their distress; five people regained their **hearing**, when she fried Green Field Onion (Ornithogalum caudatum) in Camomile oil and this warm oil was dropped into the ear frequently.

This "Camomile Witch" gave movement back to **paralyzed limbs** through Camomile oil massages. Against **eye-pain** Camomile boiled in milk was applied as a compress over the closed eyes which healed in a short time. And the Abbé Kuenzle goes on: "A weaver could only sleep sitting up; he thought he would suffocate. The herb woman took a look at him and said he was **not passing water** which he acknowledged. Immediately he had to drink from a large bottle of wine in which Camomile had been boiled, a glassful mornings and evenings. An unbelievable amount of urine was passed; first dark and turgid, then clearer and clearer and after 8 days he was healed."

DIRECTIONS

Infusion: A heaped teaspoon to ¼ litre of water, infused for a short time.

Bath addition: For a full bath use 2 double handfuls, for facial and hair wash 1 handful of Camomile flowers, pour boiling water over them and infuse.

Compress: ¼ litre of boiling milk is poured over a heaped tablespoon of Camomile, infused for a short time, strained and used warm.

Inhalation: 1 litre of boiling water is poured over a heaped tablespoon of Camomile. The steam is inhaled under a towel.

Herb pillow: A linen bag is filled with loosely dried Camomile flowers and stitched up; warmed in a dry pan and used.

Camomile oil: A small bottle is filled loosely with fresh Camomile flowers picked in the sun and cold-pressed olive-oil is poured in until it covers the flowers. The bottle, well stoppered, is kept in the sun for 14 days. Store in the refrigerator.

Camomile ointment: 250 gm. of lard are heated, one heaped double handful of fresh Camomile flowers are added; as it foams it is stirred, removed from the stove, covered and kept in a cool place overnight. Next day it is warmed and pressed through a piece of linen. The best way to do this is to place a sieve with a piece of linen inside over a jug or pot with a spout, strain and squeeze out the last bit of lard. The ointment mass is stirred and filled into clean glass jars or pots.

COLTSFOOT (Tussilago farfara)

Common names: Horsehoof, Coughwort, Bull's Foot and Foalswort.

When our meadows and hills show no sign of spring and the eye just barely notices the swelling of the willow-catkins, the Coltsfoot is the first to appear, sending forth its stalk with the yellow flower.

Wet ground, embankments, wasteland and gravel-pits are covered with blankets of Coltsfoot flowers, which appear long before the leaves. Coltsfoot grows especially well on clay soil. Bees and insects visit it to get their first nectar. These are the first flowers that can be gathered to lay in stock for the coming winter. With its pectoral and anti-inflammatory qualities Coltsfoot is used successfully for **bronchitis, laryngitis, pharyngitis, bronchial asthma and pleurisy**, even at the onset of **tuberculosis** of the lungs. For a persistent **cough** and for annoying **hoarseness** Coltsfoot tea with honey should be drunk very hot frequently during the day.

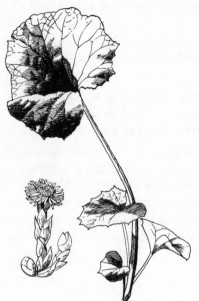

Later in May, when the leaves appear green on the upper surface and silvery felted beneath, they are used, because rich in vitamin C, as an addition to soups and salads. Since the leaves have more medicinal power than the flowers, they are gathered to be used together with the flowers for infusions.

From ancient herbalists to the Abbé Kneipp, all give praise to the Coltsfoot. The fresh leaves, washed and the pulp applied as a poultice to the chest, help in **pneumonia, in erysipelas and bruises** with swelling and discolouration and even **bursitis**. The effect of these poultices is startling. Compresses made from a strong decoction of the leaves of Coltsfoot are used for **scrofulous sores**. The steam of Coltsfoot, from the flowers as well as from the leaves, should be inhaled several times a day in chronic **bronchitis** with fits and **shortness of breath. Swollen feet** should be bathed in a decoction made of the leaves of Coltsfoot.

A syrup, prepared from the leaves, has proved its worth in **lung disorders and bronchitis**. In an earthenware pot put alternate layers of leaves and raw sugar, let it settle and keep adding until the pot is full. Cover well with 2 to 3 layers of strong parchment paper. Now put the pot in a hole in the ground in a sheltered spot in the garden. Place a board over it and cover with soil. The even temperature produces fermentation. After 8 weeks dig out the pot, boil up the syrup thus obtained, once or twice. Pour into small wide necked bottles. This syrup is our best protection against winter and influenza. Take it in teaspoonful doses.

For **asthma, damage caused by smoking and bronchitis**, 2 to 3 teaspoons of freshly pressed juice of the leaves taken in a cup of broth or warm milk, are beneficial.

For **phlebitis**, a poultice, prepared from the crushed leaves and fresh cream, is applied to the inflamed areas and bandaged lightly with a cloth. The freshly pressed juice from the leaves of the Coltsfoot is dropped into the ear to relieve **earache**.

Cough infusion: For a tea that is an expectorant; mix equal parts of the leaves and flowers of Coltsfoot, Lungwort and Plantain. Take 2 teaspoons of this mixture to ¼ litre of boiling water. Sip 3 cups of this tea sweetened with honey daily.

DIRECTIONS

Infusion: A heaped teaspoon of flowers (later equal parts of flowers and leaves) per ¼ litre boiling water, infuse for a short time.

Poultice: Fresh leaves are crushed and applied.

Inhalation: A heaped tablespoon of flowers and leaves, infuse and inhale the steam under a towel. Repeat several times a day.

Foot bath: A heaped double handful of leaves is infused in the appropriate amount of water for a short time; bathe for 20 minutes.

Fresh juice: Washed fresh leaves are put in a juice extractor.

Syrup and infusion for cough and hoarseness: Refer to part in above text.

COMFREY (Symphytum officinale)

Common names: Knit Bone, Boneset, Consound and Bruise wort.

This medicinal plant belongs to our most indispensable and valued herbs, which nature has in store for us. It grows in moist meadows, ditches and near streams, is found also near fences and in gravel pits, flowering all summer. The leaves are rough and pointed at the end. The several year old root, dark brown

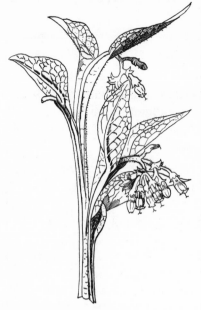

to black on the outside, white to yellowish within, is of the thickness of a thumb and, cut open, is sticky, almost slimy. The root is dug out in spring or autumn. The fresh plant is gathered before and during the time of flowering.

The tincture of Comfrey, easily prepared, contains wonderful power. People, who suffer from **rheumatism and swelling of joints** and have been treated with other remedies without success, have found relief with Comfrey tincture. A woman could hardly use her right arm (the socket joint was almost unusable) and the doctor had already diagnosed paralysis. Following my advice, she rubbed the tincture into the joint of the right arm daily. From day to day she felt how her complaint eased. Today she can use her arm normally and can look after her household. The leaves of Comfrey, scalded and used as a poultice and applied to **paralyzed limbs** caused by **over exertion, dislocation, sprain or shock**, help overnight.

My husband's aunt was hit by a motorcycle. She was taken to the hospital with a fracture of the hip joint; a pin was inserted and after she was cured, she left the hospital. After a year the pin should have been removed but since she had no pain and could walk soundly, she refrained from going to the arranged check-up. Everything seemed in good order, until one day she felt unbearable pain. The pin had to be removed and it was found that the **bone** was **infected**. Injections dulled the pain for short periods, but the infections did not heal. In this state she came to visit us, a picture of misery. I can state without exaggeration that warm poultices of Comfrey helped overnight. Next day the woman was able to sit and lie without pain. Since only small pieces of Comfrey roots were available in herbal shops, the clever aunt dried them a little more in the oven and ground them with a coffee grinder (a poppyseed grinder does it as well). She applied these poultices (see "directions") until she had no more complaints.

Knobs on the joints of hands and feet are made to disappear with these poultices. I would like to point out that the Comfrey meal itself, applied as a poultice, gives ease in **paraplegia**. Warm poultices are helpful in **varicose ulcers, muscular rheumatism, gout stones, ulcers, neck pains, painful amputation stumps, and periostitis** itself.

A tea can be prepared from the roots and used internally for **bronchitis, disorders of the digestive system, bleeding in the stomach and pleurisy**. 2 to 4 cups are sipped during the day. For **stomach ulcers** a tea of 100 gm. Comfrey, 50 gm. Calendula and 50 gm. Knot grass (Polygnom aviculare) is recommended (see "directions").

Once again I would like to mention the Comfrey tincture. As a compress it is used most successfully for external and internal **wounds**, all sorts of **injuries, bruises, contusions, ecchymosis and bone fractures**.

The leaves of Comfrey are not only used as poultices but also as additions to baths for **rheumatic complaints, gout, painful bones, slipped discs and defective circulation**.

For defective circulation in the legs, varicose veins and as supplementary treatment of **bone fractures**, Comfrey sitz baths are taken.

In an old German recipe Comfrey leaves are dipped into a light batter and fried in oil. There is goodness there for the whole family.

DIRECTIONS

Tea preparation from the roots: 2 teaspoons of finely chopped roots are soaked in ¼ litre cold water overnight, slightly warmed in the morning, strained and taken in sips.

Tea (for stomach ulcers): A heaped teaspoon of the mixture (see text above) to ¼ litre of boiling water, infuse for 3 minutes. 3 to 4 cups are sipped during the day.

Poultice: Well dried roots are finely ground, mixed quickly with very hot water and a few drops of cooking oil and spread on a piece of linen, applied warm on the affected area and bandaged.

DIRECTIONS (Comfrey)

Leaf applications (fresh): Fresh leaves are washed, beaten to a pulp and applied to the affected part.

Leaf applications (hot): Comfrey leaves are scalded and applied warm.

Additions to full bath: 500 gm. fresh or dried Comfrey leaves are soaked in approx. 5 litres of cold water. Next day it is brought to the boil and the liquid is added to the bath water (see "full bath" – General Information).

Sitz bath: Proceed as for full bath, but use only 200 gm. of leaves.

Comfrey tincture: Comfrey roots are washed and cleaned with a brush, finely chopped, loosely placed in a bottle, rye whisky or wodka poured over them and the bottle kept in the sun or near the stove for 14 days.

Comfrey ointment: 4 to 6 fresh, washed Comfrey roots, depending on size, are finely chopped and added to 250 gm. of heated lard and left to cool overnight. Next day reheated, lightly strained and pressed through a cloth, immediately poured into clean, small jars and stored in the refrigerator. This Comfrey ointment can be used instead of the meal. For treatment of wounds in humans and animals the ointment is invaluable.

Comfrey wine: 2 to 5 fresh roots are finely chopped and macerated in one litre of white wine for 5 to 6 weeks. An excellent remedy for pulmonary complaints!

COMMON CLUB MOSS (Lycopodium clavatum)

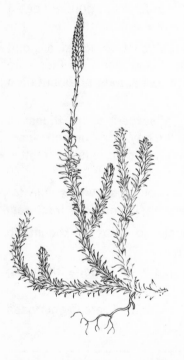

Common names: Vegetable Sulphur and Wolf's Claw.

This mossy evergreen plant has 1 to 2 metre long ramblers which trail along the forest ground with their hair-like roots. From these ramblers grow 7 to 10 cm. high forked branches soft to the touch. The 4 year old plants develop yellowish spikes which yield the pollen, called Club Moss powder, which is homoepathically employed for excoriated surfaces of the skin.

The Club Moss is a radium containing plant and easily distinguished by its widely ranging, rope-like ramblers and the yellow pollen of the spikes. It is found all over the world and occurs in high forests on Northern slopes and in moors. If the forests are cut down, the plant turns yellow and shrivels up, since it looses its life force through the direct sunlight.

For **gout and rheumatism**, even if the **joints are deformed, for chronic constipation and piles**, Club Moss tea is recommended. However, people who suffer from diarrhoea should use the tea only with the greatest caution as cramps in the intestines could develop. Club Moss is never boiled, water is poured over it. The tea is useful for all **complaints of the urinary- and reproductive organs, for inflammations and hardening of the testes, formation of gravel in the kidneys and renal colic**. For inflammation of the liver, **growth of the connective tissues of the liver**, even if malignant, Club Moss is indispensable. With its use the convalescent quickly regains his strength.

The husband of an acquaintance of mine suffered for years from **shortness of breath** at night which was treated as asthma. It got worse until one day he visited the doctor again. "If you don't stop working immediately you'll be a dead man in a week." The doctor transferred him to a hospital in my hometown. From his wife I learned that he suffered from **hardening of the liver (cirrhosis of the liver)** in its last state. Shortness of breath at night is one symptom of it. After a time he was sent home, a doomed man. On my advice the woman got some Club Moss which helped very quickly. Don't you think it a miracle if I tell you that this man lost his terrible nightly shortness of breath after his first cup of Club Moss tea?

If you know someone in your circle of friends suffering from **cirrhosis of the liver**, even if it is very bad, give this person hope and point to our radium containing Club Moss so important in herbal medicine.

During a walking tour through the forest which I undertook with a small group of people in Upper Austria, I pointed out to the Botanist, Dr. Bruno Weinmeister, the medicinal value of Club Moss in regard to cirrhosis and cancer of the liver. He thereupon told of the following event: As a young student he and his friends had been walking in the mountains. On the path to the hut between dwarfpines he found a Club Moss rambler. In high spirits, he wound it around his hat. In the hut one of his friends got a terrible **cramp in his foot**, that is, the foot stood at an angle to the knee. Everyone tried to help. The hutkeeper brought "Franzbranntwein" (an embrocation made of diluted spirits of wine and essence) and massaged the foot without success. Following a suggestion, the young Weinmeister wound the Club Moss around the cramped foot up to the knee. In a moment the foot turned back to its normal position. Now he thought this was a coincidence. Perhaps the cramp would have gone without the Club Moss. On the way home he picked a handful of Club Moss for his landlady who suffered from **leg cramps**. These brought the lady immediate relief. A few years later, Dr. Weinmeister talked about this incident to a specialist and learned from him that the Common Club Moss is a radium containing plant. Since then many people have been cured of **cramps in the legs and feet** with the help of a Club Moss pillow.

A friend was taken to hospital since she could not urinate. The upper arm was quite swollen. After she had left the hospital it started again and was as before. Luckily I had some Club Moss at home, as my mother-in-law — her age at that time was 86 years — suffered from cramps in her legs. My assumption that my friend suffered from a **cramp in her bladder** was confirmed when I applied a small bag of dried Club Moss to the region of the bladder and in a few minutes she was able to urinate normally. This small bag of Club Moss she kept applied to the region of the bladder for a few more days.

I myself suffered from **high blood pressure** for years. Mostly this was due to overfunctioning of the kidneys. Therefore I applied a small bag stuffed with Club Moss to the kidney region overnight. The next day my blood pressure was down from 200 to 165. Since then I apply a small bag filled with Club Moss to the kidney region from time to time.

For **cramps in the leg**, the Club Moss is placed in a cloth and tied around the calf. Foot baths can be taken, and also sitz baths for **cramps in the bladder** (see General Information "sitz bath").

War and accident injuries leave scars which sometimes cause cramps. A disabled soldier had a large scar on his back. This scar gave him from time to time terribly painful cramps which caused heavy perspiration all over. The pain spread over his scalp. Through the use of the Club Moss pillow and baths I was able to relieve this man's pain of 30 years duration.

The Club Moss powder, also sold as "Club Moss Spores", heals **bedsores** of seriously ill people in a short time. The Club Moss powder is finely and gently spread over the **open sores**. Generally there is a noticeable relief after the first use.

DIRECTIONS

Infusion: ¼ litre of boiling water is poured over a level teaspoon of Club Moss, infused for a short time. Only 1 cup is taken in sips on an empty stomach, half an hour before breakfast. For cirrhosis and malignant diseases of the liver, 2 cups are drunk daily.

Club Moss Pillow: Dried Club Moss (100 gm., 200 gm. or 300 gm. depending on the size of the area affected by a cramp) is stuffed into a pillow which is applied to the aching area overnight. This pillow retains its effect for one year.

Sitz bath: See "General Information", page 8.

COWSLIP (Primula officinalis)

Common names: Herb Peter, Key Flower, Key of Heaven, Fairy Cups and Paigles. — The golden yellow blossoms of this variety of Cowslip have an honey-like, agreeable fragrance and, forming an umbel on a long stalk, rise out of the centre of a rosette of leaves. It is found mostly on mountain slopes and pastures.

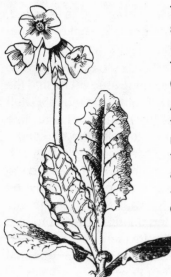

The "**tall Cowslip**" (Primula elatior), which is found abundantly in the countryside, carries on its long stem light yellow flowers with only a light fragrance. Both have the same medicinal value and can be used in the same way.

The third variety **Auriculus** (Primula auricula) is a frequent garden plant in Great Britain, though native to the Alps, where it is protected.

At a dinner I sat next to a gentleman who was taking the waters nearby. This treatment had been his last hope but now that it was drawing to a close and no improvement in his health was in sight, he was at his wit's end. Despite taking strong sleeping pills he could not find sleep. As soon as he lay down, a pain — as if someone was stubbing out a cigarette on the sole of his foot — shot through him. He felt close to a nervous breakdown. I told him I knew of an excellent tea for **insomnia**. But would it help him, he who had taken sleeping pills for so long? He tried it. It was on the 7th of December, 1976 when we met. Seven days later I met some of his friends who told me that our common friend could sleep again. At the same time he had lost the pain in his feet. The tea had helped in such a short time, given him back his health and taken away the **nervous disorder**. His physician asked him for the recipe of the **special tea for insomnia**:

50 gm. Cowslip 25 gm. Lavender 10 gm. St. John's Wort 15 gm. Hops cones 5 gm. Valerian roots	Over one heaped teaspoonful of this blend pour ¼ litre of boiling water and infuse for 3 minutes. Drink this tea very warm, sip by sip, before going to sleep; if required, sweeten with a little honey.

This tea should be preferred to all chemical sleep inducing remedies. Sleeping pills destroy the nervous system, whereas the tea removes **nervous complaints**.

My mother gathered Cowslips every spring, because she knew how soothing they are for the **heart and nerves**. Pick only the umbel. Through its **blood cleansing** properties, it rids the body of the toxic substances which lead to **gout and rheumatic illnesses**.

The Abbé Kneipp was a great supporter of Cowslip; a painting shows him holding a Cowslip. He said: "He who has a tendency to rheumatism and gout, should drink 1 to 2 cups of Cowslip tea daily over a long period. The intense pain will slacken and with time disappear."

Cowslip tea is of value in strengthening the heart and nerves, eases the pain of **migraine** and **nervous headaches**, is excellent for **inflammation of the heart muscle, dropsy and tendency to stroke**. A decoction of the roots, mixed with honey, makes a good tea for the **kidneys**, helping to expel **stones in the bladder**.

Recommended is the following **blood purifying "spring tea"**:	
50 gm. Cowslip 50 gm. Elder flower shoots 15 gm. Stinging nettle 15 gm. Dandelion roots	Take one heaped teaspoon of this mixture to ¼ litre of boiling water, infuse for 3 minutes. May be sweetened with a little honey.
(Elder flower shoots are the cluster of flowers in their unopened green state.)	

An excellent remedy for **heart complaint** is Cowslip wine, which can be prepared in spring. A 2 litre bottle is loosely filled with fresh flowers of Cowslip (whole umbels) and pure white wine is poured over it. The flowers have to be covered. The bottle is kept, loosely stoppered, in the sun for 14 days. For heart complaints, take a sip of this wine when needed. People with a heart disease should take three tablespoonfuls a day.

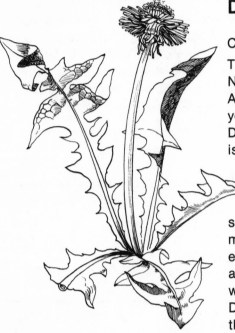

DANDELION (Taraxacum officinale)

Common names: Priest's Crown, Blow-Ball and Swine's Snout.

This plant, looked upon as a troublesome weed in lawns, is Nature's greatest healing aid for suffering mankind. It flowers in April and May in meadows and grasslands. It forms blankets of yellow flowers which turn many a place into a beautiful sight. Dandelion shuns wet places. It has two outstanding qualities: it is useful in **disorders of the liver and of the gallbladder**.

Gather the leaves before, the stems during, the time of flowering, the roots in early spring or in the autumn. The whole plant has medicinal powers. I myself have made it a habit in spring to serve the whole plant as a salad or to make an evening meal of the leaves mixed with potatoes and garnished with boiled eggs. While on a cure in Jugoslavia I noticed the guests received a small bowl of Dandelion greens besides the fresh salads. Asked why, the physician, a well-known liver specialist, told me that the Dandelion has a beneficial effect on the liver. Today I know that the fresh stems of the flower, five to six pieces, chewed daily bring swift relief in **chronic inflammation of the liver** (sharp pain felt in the region of the lower corner of the right shoulderblade). As long as the plant is in flower, **diabetics** should eat up to 10 stems daily. The stems with the flowers are washed and only then is the flowerhead removed and the stems are slowly chewed. They taste somewhat bitter at first, but are crisp and juicy similar to a leaf of endive. Sickly people who feel constantly tired and are without energy should take a 14-day course of treatment with the fresh stems of Dandelion. The effect is surprising.

But in many more troubles they are of value; in **itchy and scaly rashes and eczema**. The flow of **gastric juices** is improved and the stomach is cleaned of all waste matter. The fresh stems can help remove **gall stones** painlessly — they **stimulate the liver** and the **gallbladder**.

Besides mineral salts, Dandelion contains active substances which are of value in **metabolic disturbances**. As a **blood purifier** it brings relief in **gout and rheumatism, glandular swellings** subside if a 3- to 4-week course of treatment with the fresh stems is adhered to. For **jaundice and disorders of the spleen**, Dandelion is also used successfully.

Dandelion roots, eaten raw or taken dry in the form of an infusion, **purify the blood, improve digestion** and have a **diuretic, sudorific** as well as a **stimulating effect**.

Old herbals state that women used the infusion of the plant and roots as a **beauty aid** and washed their **faces and eyes** with it, hoping to gain youthful looks. The leaves keep growing even in the cold time of the year.

Every year in spring I prepare **syrup from the flowers of Dandelion** which not only tastes good but at the same time is wholesome. My Christmas ginger biscuits are all made with this syrup.

My mother once met a woman, carrying an apron full of Dandelion flowers. Asked about the reason the woman gave the following recipe for the delicious syrup:

Two heaped double handfuls of Dandelion flowers are put in 1 litre of cold water and slowly brought to the boil; removed from the heat and left overnight. The next day this is strained and the flowers well pressed out. To this liquid is added 1 kilo of raw sugar and half a sliced lemon (if sprayed — use without skin). If more lemon is used, it makes it sour. The pot is put on the stove without a lid and simmered on a low heat so as not to destroy the vitamins. Test for consistency. It should neither be too thick, it would crystallize when stored for a time, nor too thin, it would sour. The right consistency is a thick-flowing syrup that, spread on a bun or on a piece of buttered bread, tastes delicious.

Once we had a carpenter working at our place and in the evening I prepared a cold meal for him, whereas my family enjoyed buttered bread with the freshly made syrup. He asked if he could try it too. As an apiarist, he did not believe that I had prepared this "honey". He was enthusiastic and he said he found hardly any difference between the honey and the syrup. I would like to add that people with kidney complaints do not tolerate well the acid in the honey whereas the Dandelion syrup is easily digested.

This valuable medicinal plant has an important place in herbal medicine. Unfortunately a large part of the populace does not recognize it and only looks upon it as a terrible weed. One day I noticed a young man whose face was covered with **acne**. I brought the blood purifying effect of the Dandelion and Stinging Nettle to his mother's attention. She did not even know the Dandelion although she was from our small town and not from a big city. When I described the plant to her she said with indignation that she could not offer such weeds to her son.

DIRECTIONS

Infusion: 1 heaped tablespoon of roots is soaked in cold water overnight, brought to the boil and strained next day. This amount is apportionately sipped, half an hour before and half an hour after breakfast.

Salad: Made from fresh roots and leaves (see above text).

Stems: 5 to 10 flower stems are well chewed and eaten daily.

Syrup: See above text.

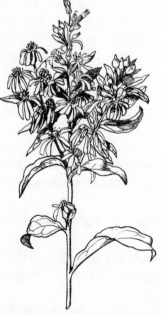

GOLDEN ROD (Solidago virga-aurea)

Common names: Solidago, Aaron's Rod.

This medicinal plant is found in woods and copses, in moist ditches and on hillsides. The erect stem with its bushy branches on the upper half, carrying yellow star-like flowers, grows to about 80 cm. The flowers are gathered from July to October and are used for disorders and **bleeding of the intestines**. Especially though, Golden Rod is praised as an excellent remedy for **disorders of the kidneys**.

Flowers and leaves of the Golden Rod have a cooling effect and, since the plant is a diuretic, are recommended in all **kidney and bladder complaints**. The Swiss herbalist, Abbé Kuenzle, tells in his writings of a 45 year old man who suffered from a serious kidney complaint which got worse and worse. Finally one kidney had to be removed. The other one was affected as well and could not work properly. This man began a Golden Rod treatment. He mixed equal parts of Golden Rod, Bedstraw and Yellow Dead Nettle, prepared a tea and sipped 3 to 4 cups during the day, whereupon he recovered, as he said himself, in 14 days.

Golden Rod together with Bedstraw and Yellow or White Dead Nettle is efficacious in cases of **cirrhosis of the kidneys and renal failure** when renal dialysis has to be performed. In these cases I was able to help, using the above mentioned herbs: A 52 year old man, suffering from cirrhosis of the kidneys, came to see me. Puffing and sweating heavily he climbed up the stairs to the first floor where I lived. Fighting for breath he fell into a chair. In a week, after having drunk 3 cups of tea made of the above mentioned herb mixture, he felt a lot better. He used only fresh herbs. After the third week he was free from complaints.

All our **emotions** are worked off through the kidneys. Therefore they are the most affected after an **emotional shock**, be it a death in the family or any other accident. Golden Rod proves its worth as a medicinal plant which influences the human emotions most favourably. It should therefore be drunk without delay in cases of **disappointments and emotional stress.**

We feel the soothing effect of this plant almost like a calming and caressing hand in **severe emotional stress.** Even the sight of the Golden Rod in nature has a quieting effect on us. We should be thankful that there grows a plant around us which can bring us such comfort.

DIRECTION

Infusion: ¼ litre of boiling water is poured over 1 heaped teaspoon of Golden Rod and infused for a short time. – One heaped teaspoon of the mixture is also used and prepared as above.

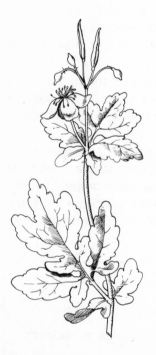

GREATER CELANDINE (Chelidonium majus)

Common names: Swallow Wort, Garden Celandine, Tetterwort, Felonwort.
Greater Celandine is not related to the Lesser Celandine (Ranunculus ficaria) and the only thing they have in common is the colour of their flowers.

Greater Celandine grows to a height of 30 to 80 cm., is much branched and flowers from May until well into Autumn. Its much-divided leaves resemble oak-leaves and the roots and stems have an orange-yellow juice. It grows in hedgerows, by walls and fences, on waste ground and favours south-facing edges of woods. The summer may be dry and the ground parched and the orange-yellow juice still flows freely when the stem is broken. Even in winter this plant can be found under the snow, if its position is known.

The plant **purifies and stimulates the blood** and I would use it together with Stinging Nettle and Elder shoots in cases of **leukaemia.** But to be effective, at least 2 litres of tea made from the mixture have to be drunk daily.

Greater Celandine is a reliable remedy for serious **liver ailments** when used in a homeopathic form. Because of its **blood** and **liver-cleansing qualities** it has a positive influence on the metabolism. This medicinal herb can be used effectively for **gall bladder, kidney and liver diseases.** Prepared with wine (30 g Greater Celandine including the roots should be placed in half a liter of white wine for one or two hours), it is a quick cure for **jaundice.** It can also be recommended for **haemorrhoids** accompanied by a burning sensation in the anus, for **stinging pain and cramps while urinating,** as well as for buzzing in the ears. In these cases 2 – 3 cups of tea (which should be scalded but not boiled) should be sipped throughout the day. Externally the juice is used for **malignant skin disorders, corns, warts and incurable herpes. Cataract and spots on the cornea** are caused to disappear gradually. The juice even helps in cases of a **bleeding or detached retina.** A leaf of the Celandine is washed and the stem of the leaf is rubbed between the wet thumb and index finger. The juice thus won is brushed gently over the closed eyes towards the corners. Although not rubbed into the eyes, they nevertheless benefit from it. This holds good for **cataract and defective vision** and is prophylactic for healthy but strained eyes. I, myself, when working until late at night finishing my correspondence feel its beneficial effect, when overtired, I fetch a leaf of Celandine from the garden and use it as described above. It is as if a mist is lifted from my eyes. A homoeopathic tincture of Celandine is used for the above mentioned disorders, in 10 to 15 drop doses, diluted in some water and taken two to three times daily.

A few year ago, I was told of a farmer's wife who had a red **growth**, the size of a little finger tip, on the lower eyelid. The eye specialist from whom she wanted a prescription for glasses did not like the look of it — she had this growth for 7 to 8 years without it causing her any pain — and obtained a biopsy. It was cancer. For the young woman it was a terrible shock — as you can well imagine. Since the family belonged to our circle of acquaintances, I was able to bring Celandine to her notice. It was February and luckily a mild winter, Celandine stays green even in winter. I told her to dig out the plant and put it in a pot to have it handy. She had to dab the affected spot with the orange-yellow juice 5 to 6 times a day. Since the growth was on the lower eyelid I told her that it was harmless to the eye. I told her also to go to the X-ray treatment once a month as the physician had ordered, although the rays do not remove **cancer-like growths**, but in fact destroy still healthy skin and often also bones. Shortly before Christmas I had the pleasure to hear that the growth had disappeared. When the woman came to see me, she hugged me at the door. The eye specialist whom she had seen before had asked her in astonishment what she had done. To her answer: "I had the monthly X-ray treatment", he replied, "if the X-ray treatments have removed the growth, it is a miracle." She then told me that she would not have been able to cope with the faces (eaten to the bone) of the other patients whom she saw when waiting for her treatment, had I not given her a lot of hope, faith and belief in herself. Now my request to you all: Do help in similar cases and save your fellow human being from a terrible end. In the environment polluting times in which we live, there is an increase in cases of **skin cancer** developing out of red and suddenly enlarging warts.

Facial hair and **increased growth of hair** on arms and legs of women points to kidney disorders. Celandine juice which is obtained with the juice extractor (the fresh juice will keep up to six months in the refrigerator) is dabbed on the affected places; it is allowed to penetrate for a few hours, then washed with a mild soap and the somewhat dried out skin is treated with Calendula ointment, Camomile oil or St. John's Wort oil (see "directions"). In addition a course of Stinging Nettle tea, at least 3 to 4 cups throughout the day, together with Horsetail sitz baths should be undertaken to better stimulate the kidneys (see under "Horsetail").

An acquaintance from the district of Mainz (Germany) used the Celandine juice as stated during his daily walks. An Alsatian dog, already on in years, was his faithful companion. As a joke he smeared the dogs eyes once with the juice which was apparently beneficial, as the dog from that time on sat begging in front of his master whenever he used the Celandine juice.

In Upper Austria, where I gave a lecture in November, I got to know a sexton who wore glasses. When I came back in February the sexton no longer wore glasses. Asked for the reason, he told me that since November he had followed my advice on the Celandine treatment daily. He **saw much better** now than before with glasses. At this time he must have obtained the Celandine leaves from beneath the snow. I cite this to show that certain medicinal plants are found fresh in winter, when all the other plants appear to be dead.

DIRECTIONS

Infusion:	¼ litre of boiling water is poured over 1 level teaspoon of herbs.
Fresh Juice:	Leaves, stems and flowers are washed and, still wet, put into the juice extractor for external application.
Tincture:	As an homoeopathic preparation bought at chemists.
Wine:	30 gm. Celandine together with roots macerated in 1 litre of white wine for 1 to 2 hours, then filter or strain and sipped.

HORSETAIL (Equisetum arvense)

Common names are Peterwort, Dutch rushes, Shave-grass and Bottle-brush. — In early spring the brown fertile stems with a terminal cone-like catkin containing the spores grow from the deep and creeping rhizomes. The green summer fronds grow later to a height of 40 cm. and resemble small, evenly built pine-trees. Horsetail grows in fields, on hedge banks and railway embankments. The ones growing on pure clay soil have the greatest healing qualities. Depending on the place it grows it has 3 to 16% of

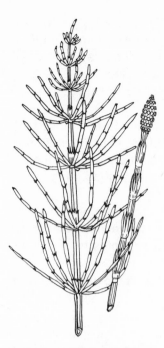

silicic acid which makes it so valuable. Of course the Horsetail growing on chemically fertilised ground should not be used. The Horsetail with the finest branches, the **Wood Horsetail** (Equisetum sylvaticum) which grows on edges of woods and copses, has medicinal properties too.

In popular medicine Horsetail was much esteemed in old times, especially for its **blood-staunching** effect and its success in **kidney and bladder trouble**. But with time its values were forgotten. It was no other than our great and popular herbalist Abbé Kneipp who put the Horsetail back to its important place. He declares it as "uniquely irreplaceable and invaluable" for **bleeding, spitting of blood, bladder- and kidney disorders, gravel and stones**. "For old troubles", he says, "**foul wounds, even cancer-like growths and ulcerated legs**, Horsetail is of great value. It cleanses, clears up and burns away everything bad, so to speak. Often the moist, warm plant is placed into moist cloths and applied to the affected parts."

The Swiss Abbé Kuenzle says that all people from a certain age on should drink a cup of Horsetail tea every day all year round and **all pain** caused by **rheumatism, gout and nerves** would **disappear** and **every person would have a healthy old age**. He tells of an 86 year old man who was relieved from stones which had caused him a lot of pain, by taking Horsetail steam baths and who still lived for many years. He also states: "This plant, taken internally as a tea, will stop the strongest **haemorrhaging** and **vomiting of blood** in a short time, yes, almost immediately."

For painful **bladder catarrh and cramp-like pains** there is no better remedy than a decoction of Horsetail, if one wraps oneself in a bath robe and allows the hot steam of the decoction to work into the bladder for 10 minutes. Repeat several times and it soon will bring relief. Old people who suddenly have **trouble urinating**, together with pain, because the urine is not expelled or does so only drop-wise, will find relief through the hot steam of Horsetail, rather than having the doctor use a catheter. For **gravel and stones in the kidney and bladder** hot Horsetail sitz baths are taken and at the same time warm Horsetail tea is sipped, the urine is held back and finally emptied under pressure. This way most stones will pass. On the strenght of this suggestion I have received letters which confirm the above: Through this treatment the **kidney stones** were passed, the persons concerned are well and without any pain.

In cases where other diuretic means failed, Horsetail helped, as for example in **accumulation of water in the pericardium, pleura, or in kidney disorders**, after scarlet fever and other bad infectious diseases with water retention. It is an excellent remedy, internally and externally, for the whole kidney and bladder system.

For **pyelitis** a bath alone can work wonders. For this can be taken – and only for **external use** – the **Great or River Horsetail** (Equisetum maximum) that grows in bogs, on banks of rivers and has finger thick stems. An acquaintance of mine was in hospital with a bad case of pyelitis for weeks. Since there seemed no end in sight, she sent a letter to me. I advised her to take a Horsetail sitz bath. A few days later I received another letter: "You have saved my life. I am at home. The sitz bath took away all troubles and gave me new strength." The Great or River Horsetail is used for sitz baths **only**. The Field or Wood Horsetail is used for teas taken internally.

After a difficult birth young mothers sometimes experience **visual defects**, the reason, most likely, is an affected kidney. Sitz baths stimulate the kidney and take the pressure off the eyes, so that slowly the visual defects disappear.

The German physician Dr. Bohn highly praises this plant: "On the one side Horsetail is a remedy for **haemorrhaging** and on the other – and even more so – a kidney remedy. After drinking the tea, a large quantity of dark coloured urine is easily passed. For **dropsy** it is a quick, effective remedy." If no other **diuretic remedy** works, all other herb teas are avoided and from 5 to 6 cups of Horsetail tea are sipped daily for 4 to 5 days (in persistent cases 6 days). Experience shows that in most cases the water passes.

For **itching rashes**, even if they are festering or scabby, washings and compresses of a decoction of Horsetail are helpful. Horsetail washings and baths are beneficial for **inflammation of the nailbed, cracked feet, caries, old festering wounds, cancer-like growths, bony projections on the heal, fistulas, barber's itch** and other **herpes**. The scalded herb, wrapped while warm in a cloth, can also be applied. For painful **haemorrhoids and haemorrhoidal knots** the pulp is used.

For persistent **nose bleeding** a compress made from the cooled decoction of Horsetail is applied. As a **blood-staunching remedy** it helps to stop **bleeding of the lung, uterus, stomach and haemorrhoids**. Of course stronger decoctions are required. Normally 1 heaped teaspoon per cup (¼ litre) is used, but for bleedings 2 to 3 heaped teaspoons per cup are required. Horsetail together with Speedwell is a good preventive remedy for **hardening of the arteries and for amnesia** through its blood cleansing action. One can call it the best cancer prophylactic.

Horsetail tincture (see "directions") is an excellent remedy for **sweaty feet**. This tincture is rubbed into the well washed and dried feet and a cup of Horsetail tea is drunk on an empty stomach half an hour before breakfast daily. Foot baths are also good for sweaty feet (see "directions"). For **dandruff**, the hair is washed with a decoction of Horsetail daily and then the scalp massaged with a good olive oil and the dandruff will soon clear up.

A tea of Horsetail and St. John's Wort — 2 cups daily and a nonliquid meal in the evening will relieve **bedwetting**. This tea can also be used as a gargle for **tonsillitis, inflammation of the mucous membrane of the mouth, stomatitis, inflammation or bleeding of the gums, fistulas and adenoids** in palate and throat. For **white discharge** in woman, sitz baths are used.

Don't forget, Horsetail is one of the best remedies for **chronic bronchitis and tuberculosis of the lungs**. Through its silica content, the tea, if drunk regularly, helps heal the lungs and removes the **general weakness**.

Results of the latest research, according to the Austrian biologist Richard Willfort, justify the assumption that **tumours** are inhibited in their growth and finally eliminated through the use of Horsetail tea for long periods. This is also useful for **polyps** in the abdomen or anus. For greater benefit in both cases Horsetail steam poultices and sitz baths are used. These poultices are also useful for **stomach pains, liver- and gallbladder attacks, bursitis** and for painful **congestions** which press upon the **heart**.

On December 19, 1977 I received a call from a 49 year old farmer, who had a very painful, hard **growth** on the sole of his foot and was therefore unable to step on it. He spent a few days in hospital but was sent home again. I recommended Horsetail poultices which can even eliminate malignant tumours. I was quite surprised when on December 22, he called again telling me that the growth had disappeared. The skin still felt soft and flabby but the hard growth was gone. — A new miracle from God's pharmacy!

I have found through experience that the worst **disc lesions** insofar as they are not caused by a pinched nerve, often disappear very quickly through the use of Horsetail sitz baths. If X-rays show degenerated vertebrae caused by age, there is no reason to suffer pain. The pressure of a kidney disorder pushes upward and along the spine where it presses on the superficial nerves causing pain, as experience shows. Therefore it is the pressure of the kidneys and not the disc lesions which causes the pain. A Horsetail sitz bath because of its deep penetration relieves the pressure.

A 38 year old woman was under treatment for **disc lesions** for 3 years, but her pains became worse, her shoulders and neck area were so stiff that she could only get out of bed in the morning with the help of a bar her husband had fixed over her bed. At this time I met her at a lecture I gave. You will be quite surprised to learn that this woman lost all her stiffness and pain after only one sitz bath. This applies also for disc lesions caused by driving a tractor. The rattling movements do not harm the discs but the kidneys and immediately there is a pressure upward which Horsetail sitz baths relieve.

A lady from Switzerland had a stiff neck for years. Every year she took a cure which gave her only limited relief. By chance I met her. Sceptically she promised to take Horsetail sitz baths. Soon I received a call and this happy lady told me that after 10 minutes in the bath all the stiffness had disappeared. As I know, it has not returned since.

The great neurologist Dr. Wagner-Jauregg said in his writings: **"two thirds of all mentally ill would not go to a mental home had they healthy kidneys."** Up to now I have been able to advise many unhappy people who, through **kidney disorders**, suffered from **depression, delusions and fits of rage** and would have ended in a mental home but for Horsetail sitz baths. For these conditions besides Yarrow and Stinging Nettle teas, a cup of Horsetail tea mornings and evenings must be drunk.

For serious **kidney disorders** with all the accompanying symptoms, fresh Horsetail sitz baths should be used, the best, as mentioned previously, being the Great or River Horsetail. A 5 litre bucketful of herbs is needed for 1 bath (see "directions" and "sitz bath" under General Information). For the sitz bath the kidney region must be under water — the bath must last 20 minutes! Do not dry yourself, but, still wet, wrap yourself in a bath robe and remain perspiring in bed for one hour. Only then, dress in dry night attire. The sitz bath water can be re-warmed and used twice.

INDIAN CORN (Zea Mays)

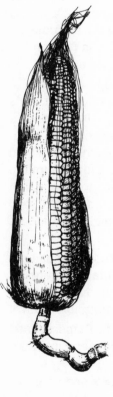

Corn is cultivated in many parts of the world and in recent years has become popular in Europe.

From the husks or ears hang many soft filaments called "the silk". This is the part that has medicinal properties. It is cut off before the pollen drops from the flowers and dried quickly in the shade.

Should a reliable **diuretic** be needed then drink Corn Silk tea which is also an effective, harmless **weight-reducer** (of interest to the many overweight people in our affluent society). If Corn Silk is stored not completely dried, it looses its diuretic qualities and becomes laxative.

For disorders of the urinary tract with formations of **stones, edema, fluid in the heart**, the Corn Silk tea is as effective as for **nephritis, cystitis, gout and rheumatism**. It can also be employed successfully in **bedwetting** of children or older people, as well as for **renal colic**. For all these disorders take one tablespoon of tea every two to three hours.

DIRECTION

Infusion: ¼ litre of hot water is poured over 1 heaped teaspoon of Corn Silk, infused for a short time, not sweetened.

LADY'S MANTLE (Alchemilla vulgaris)

Common names are Lion's Foot, Bear's Foot, Nine Hooks and Dew Cup. — It is found on grasslands, woodlands, high-lying ground and in mountainous regions. The plant has somewhat kidney-shaped leaves cut into 7 to 9 shallow lobes, on stout, short stalks and inconspicuous yellowish green flowers which can be seen from April to June but often later. Some of the leaves lie flat on the ground and in the morning dewdrops can be found in the centre, shimmering like pearls. At altitudes over 1000 metres the Alchemilla alpine or Silver Lady's Mantle is found which grows on limestone as well as basalt. Gather, of both plants, the whole plant during the time of flowering, later only the leaves, and dry them in the attic. As the name implies, it is essentially a woman's herb and esteemed as such. Since Christian times it has been associated with the Virgin Mary.

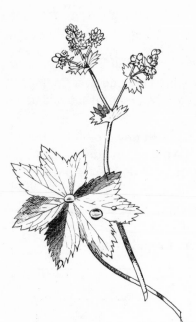

Not only is Lady's Mantle beneficial for **menstrual disorders, "whites", abdominal disorders and indisposition during menopause**, but it also helps at the beginning of **puberty**, together with Yarrow tea, to influence the onset of menstruation favourably. In cases, where, for young girls, menstruation will not commence despite professional medication, it is Lady's Mantle together with Yarrow (mixed in equal proportions) that brings everything into line. The action of Lady's Mantle is astringent and very rapid healing, and it is used also as a diuretic and heart strengthening remedy for **wound-fever**, for **festering wounds and neglected sores**. After **removal of teeth**, Lady's Mantle tea is recommended as one of the best remedies. Within a day the wounds heal after several rinses. It relieves **weakness of muscles** and limbs and helps in **anaemia (anemia).**

For **injuries after delivery, debility of the abdomen** of women who have difficult confinements or are **inclined to miscarry, for strengthening** of the foetus and **uterus**, Lady's Mantle is of great help. Women so affected should start drinking Lady's Mantle tea after the third month. It is a cure-all for all **female disorders** and, together with Shepherd's Purse, even helps in **prolapse of the uterus and in hernia**. For the last named cases, use four cups of Lady's Mantle tea, which should, as far as possible, be prepared from freshly picked herbs, and sip throughout the day. In addition, the affected parts are massaged with Shepherd's Purse tincture (see "directions" for Shepherd's Purse); for prolapse of the uterus, the massage is upward from the vagina. Additionally, Yarrow tea sitz baths (100 gm. of herbs per bath; in all three baths weekly, as the bath water, re-warmed, can be used twice).

Our forefathers used the plant as a wound herb, externally and internally, for **epilepsy and hernia**. A quotation from an old herbal says: "When one is ill, whether young or old, let two handfuls of Lady's Mantle in a measure of water boil for as long as it takes to hard boil an egg, and drink it." In today's herbal medicine the plant has again its proper place. The Swiss Abbé Kuenzle stresses its merits: "Through early and prolonged application of this medicinal herb two thirds of all operations performed on women would be quite unnecessary, since it heals all **inflammations of the abdomen, fever, burning, suppuration, ulcers and hernia**. Every woman in childbed should drink much of this tea, some children would still have their mother, some stricken widower his wife, had they but known this herb. Crushed and applied externally, Lady's Mantle heals **wounds, stings and cuts**. Children who, despite good food, have **weak muscles**, become strong through the continued use of this tea."

Alchemilla alpine, a mountain variety, has leaves with a silvery underside. It should be used in cases of **obesity**. 2 to 3 cups drunk daily, are beneficial. It is effective also for **restless nights; diabetics** should drink it often. Weak children visibly strengthen, if Lady's Mantle or, better still, Silvery Lady's Mantle is added to the bath water. For 1 bath approx. 200 gm. of herbs are used (see General Information "bath").

Lady's Mantle, together with Sherpherd's Purse, as written in full detail under Shepherd's Purse, is used for **muscular atrophy** and serious and **incurable disorders of the muscles**. This valuable medicinal herb is used for **multiple sclerosis** as well.

I have been told by people from Burgenland (Austria) that, if Lady's Mantle tea is drunk and used externally to wash the heart region, it brings a marked relief in **disorders of the cardiac muscle**.

DIRECTIONS

Infusion: ¼ litre of boiling water is poured over a heaped teaspoon of herbs, infused for a short time.

Herb application: A suitable amount of fresh herbs is washed and crushed on a wooden board with a wooden rolling pin and applied.

Bath: For a full bath, 200 gm. of dried or a few double handfuls of fresh herbs are soaked in a bucketful of cold water overnight, warmed the next morning and the liquid added to the bath water (see General Information "bath").

MALLOW (Malva vulgaris)

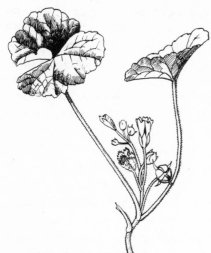

Common name is Cheeses.

The small leaved Mallow grows on old walls, near paths and on waste ground, always in the neighbourhood of human habitation. Should it be found far from it, it indicates that once a house stood there.

The large leaved Mallow – **Malva grandifolia** – and other varieties are mostly found growing in flower and vegetable gardens. Both plants contain mucilage and tannin in leaves, flowers and stems. The small leaved Mallow is somewhat creeping and slightly woody near the root stock. It has long-stemmed, round toothed leaves and small purple to pale pink flowers. The roundish fruit is called popularly "cheeses". Most country children will have eaten – and played with these "cheeses". The flowers, leaves and stems are gathered from June to September. Since, through drying, mucilage is lost, it is best to use Mallow as fresh as possible. But the dry plant still has medicinal properties.

Mallow tea is especially useful for **inflammations of the mucous membranes** throughout the body – such as the **bladder, gastro-intestinal tract and mouth** – for **gastritis**, as well as for **ulcers in the stomach and the intestines**. For this the leaves, together with barley, are made into a soup. First the barley is cooked and when cooled, the Mallow leaves are added.

It is especially recommended for **phlegm in the lungs, bronchitis, coughs and hoarseness**, as well as for **laryngitis, tonsillitis and dry mouth**. So as not to destroy the mucilage in the plant, the Mallow is soaked in cold water overnight. 2 to 3 cups of the slightly warmed tea are sipped throughout the day. Even for stubborn and, as often represented, incurable **emphysema** which causes difficult breathing, it is effective. At least 3 cups are drunk per day and the strained and warmed leaves and flowers are applied as a poultice on the chest overnight.

Especially beneficial are eyewashes and eye compresses of the lukewarm Mallow tea for the rarely occurring drying up of the **tear ducts**.

Washings with the lukewarm Mallow tea are soothing in cases of **allergies in the face**, which cause itching and burning. Externally, Mallow is used for **wounds, ulcers, swollen feet and hands**, which result from **fractures or phlebitis**. In these cases hand or foot baths are taken (see "directions").

I have had great success with these baths. For a **fracture** of the foot bone, where the foot is again and again overburdened and swells up, Mallow baths are to be specially recommended.

In our neighbourhood lives a woman who broke her ankle joint a few years ago. She had constant difficulties with her foot and one day the woman had to return to hospital. I met her after her discharge from the hospital, the foot and leg swollen to above the knee. Although she used a stick, she only came forward at a snail's pace. We gathered fresh Mallow. On the next day the woman began with the foot baths. I do not exaggerate when I relate that after one week she no longer needed the stick, and the foot looked normal again; likewise for another woman with a broken right wrist that caused her difficulties again and again. Which housewife and mother can spare her right hand? Every night the hand throbbed and for a long time it swelled daily. When I met her, I recommended Mallow. In this case as well, it became better very quickly.

A **swollen, open foot**, even when one is old, is really not necessary. Mallow baths, together with fresh Plantain leaves, help here too. The latter, well washed and still wet, are laid on the open wound. The wound closes overnight and does not open again, even if the wound is 10 to 15 years old or much older. Should you suffer from such open wounds, then follow my advice on the fresh Plantain leaves. You will be surprised how quickly the wounds close. And when reading these lines, do not think: "Mrs. Treben has overstepped the mark this time!" I can only relate what I have been able to gather from my experiences.

Now I will relate a story, that sounds wonderful, yet is true. It is astonishing, what this tiny creeping medicinal herb accomplishes. One day I sat alone at a table in a restaurant in Linz. A woman joined me; from the conversation I learned that she had the greatest concern for her husband who had to go to hospital from time to time and had now lost his voice. The doctors always avoided her questions so that at last she feared that it was **cancer of the larynx**. "Dont give up hope", I said. "Try the medicinal herbs. We have the valuable Mallow, which helps with **inflammation of the larynx**. One gargles with it frequently during the day and uses the tea residue – mixed with barley flour – as a warm poultice overnight." This was on a Thursday. We had become really friendly and exchanged addresses. In the following week on Wednesday I received a telephone call from this lady. "My husband is already better. We have done everything, as you said. I have a daughter who is a doctor in Vienna. I told her of my plan to take her father out of the hospital and try medicinal herbs. 'If it comforts you mother, do it', she said. At the same time I spoke to our specialist who said likewise that he was not against herbs in principle. So I brought my husband home; he gargled and I made him the warm poultices for his throat. A few days ago he had his voice back." A week later came a second call: "My husband is well. He is very hopeful that he can take up teaching again shortly. I would like to tell you, what the specialist said, when I told him all about it: 'This woman deserves a gold medal!'"

Our good Mallow not only takes away **inflammation of the larynx**, but also malignant **larynx disorders**. In such cases, use 2½ litres as the daily ration steeped overnight (one heaped teaspoon of herbs per ¼ litre). In the morning, warm slightly and the prescribed quantity is kept in a thermos flask, rinsed with hot water. Throughout the day, 4 cups are sipped, the rest is used for gargling. For **dryness in the mouth, throat and nose**, which often makes the patients very nervous, Mallow tea is used frequently as a gargle and rinse throughout the day.

In our time the Mallow which grows mainly by farmhouses, is disappearing more and more. In an attempt to keep moisture and dirt away from the house and to give the outside a nice appearance, a cement strip or a gutter is often laid around the house. Thus the Mallow is prevented from growing in its ancestral location. In this way Man's great helper disappears.

DIRECTIONS

Infusion: Only cold infusions! A heaped teaspoon of herbs per ¼ litre of water is soaked overnight, slightly warmed in the morning.

Foot and hand baths: A heaped double handful of Mallow soaked in a 5 litre container of cold water overnight. The next day it is warmed so that hands and feet can stand it. Bathe for 20 minutes. It can be used twice more.

Poultice: The residue of the tea preparation is slightly warmed in some water, mixed with barley flour, spread on a piece of linen and applied warm.

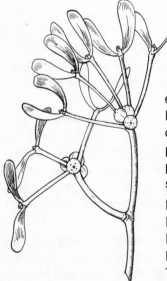

MISTLETOE (Viscum album)

Common names: European Mistletoe and Birdlime Mistletoe.

The well-known Mistletoe, an evergreen, parasitic plant, grows on deciduous trees and pine trees in a ball-like bush and is an excellent medicinal herb one should not do without. The evergreen, leathery leaves are of a yellow-green colour. The berries are whitish, somewhat opaque and sticky. Birds distribute the sticky seeds in this way: by sharpening their beaks on branches or passing the undigested seeds in droppings. Only in this way is it propagated since it has been demonstrated that seeds do not sprout when placed either in water or soil.

Mistletoe, an old magic and medicinal plant, is shrouded in mystery. The Druids held it in great reverence as a sacred plant that could remove every ill. It was gathered with great ceremony and cut from the tree with a golden knife. Old herbalists used it as an excellent and effective remedy for **epilepsy**. This remedy is also acknowledged by the "Kneipp" physician, Dr. Bohn. He recommends Mistletoe for **chronic cramps and hysterical complaints**.

The leaves and small twigs which are cut for drying are gathered from the beginning of October to the middle of December and then in March and April. In the remaining months of the year, Mistletoe is without medicinal properties. Plants with the greatest healing power grow on oaks and poplars; but those growing on pines, firs and fruit trees are also medicinally strong. Again a hint on gathering: In March and April the Mistletoe has hardly any berries. The birds have picked them in winter. There is less work then in cutting the leaves and twigs, since the removal of the sticky berries that are still there between October and December is no longer necessary.

Frequently I have been asked why I praise Mistletoe so much, since it is supposed to be poisonous. The leaves and twigs are not; only the berries, if taken internally. An ointment made of the berries and lard is excellent for **frost bites** (see "directions").

A woman had **chilblains** on her nose for years. During winter she was reluctant to leave the house because of her blue-red nose. It got worse from year to year. I advised her to apply a poultice of fresh Mistletoe berries on her nose overnight. Although it sounds unbelievable it is a fact that her nose was normal after a few days.

Since Mistletoe benefits the whole **glandular system** it also aids the **metabolism**. At the same time it favourably influences the **pancreas** so that through drinking Mistletoe tea over a long period, **diabetes** loses its original cause. Especially people who suffer from **chronic metabolic disorders** should try to drink Mistletoe tea regularly for six months. It is excellent for **hormonal imbalance**. In this case at least 2 cups a day, one in the morning and one in the evening, are sipped.

For **hardening of the arteries** Mistletoe is an excellent remedy, esteemed and recommended for **stroke**, which would scarcely have happened, had the tea been drunk regularly. After a stroke drink 3 cups a day for 6 weeks, 2 cups for 3 weeks and 1 cup for 2 weeks; the first cup, half before and half after breakfast, the second cup before and after lunch and the third cup before and after dinner.

Mistletoe tea is also used as a **blood-staunching** remedy. It stops **nose-bleeding** when used cold, if drawn up into the nose. As a tea it arrests **lung- and intestines-bleeding** caused by **typhoid or dysentery**.

Mistletoe is the best remedy for **heart and circulatory** complaints. I cannot emphasize Mistletoe enough for circulatory problems. Since it has active substances which normalize the whole system, it lowers **high** and raises **low blood pressure**. It soothes the restless heart and strengthens it. All the side effects of abnormal blood pressure such as **blood rushing to the head, dizziness, buzzing in the ears and visual defects** disappear. Mistletoe, it can be said, is invaluable in all **heart and circulatory disorders**. People in our fast moving times, with the tensions of modern living and working under stress, surely need an aid like Mistletoe.

In many letters I have received, people state that thanks to Mistletoe they have found relief in a short time from **high blood pressure, bad circulatory problems, lack of energy, heart disorders, heart flutters, dizziness and unwillingness to work**. 3 cups of Mistletoe, made as a cold infusion and sipped throughout the day, will normalize your heart and your circulation and guarantee an increased work activity. In general, Mistletoe tea should be drunk for six weeks, once a year; 3 cups for 3 weeks, 2 cups for 2 weeks and 1 cup for 1 week. Blood pressure and circulation will have recovered after this. To keep it that way it is of benefit to keep on drinking 1 cup in the morning for a year.

A gentleman from the district of Mainz (Germany) suffered from **low blood pressure** for years, sometimes so badly he was unable to work. He had tried different doctors, but still he was no better. He was very sceptical about my advice that Mistletoe lowers high blood pressure and raises low blood pressure. It was April and the Mistletoe still had its healings powers. A few months later, during a talk I gave in Upper Austria, he sat in the first row and told everyone that now his blood pressure was normal.

Women, too, should take Mistletoe tea. The normalized circulation brings **uterine and menstrual disorders** into equilibrium, especially heavy **menstruation** as well as bleeding after confinement. For **palpitations of the heart, difficulties in breathing, hot flushes and feelings of anxiety during menopause**, Mistletoe tea, drunk for a few years, brings relief and you will pass through the change naturally. The fresh juice of Mistletoe, 25 drops in water on an empty stomach before breakfast and 25 drops in water in the evening before going to bed will remedy **barreness** in woman.

Some time ago an announcement appeared in the London press that three independently working research groups came to the conclusion that a high percentage of women over 50 years of age developed cancer of the breast, if they have, for treatment of high blood pressure, taken blood pressure reducing medication over a long period. Why take this risk, when we have our valuable Mistletoe?

Lately, Mistletoe is used medicinally to **counteract and prevent cancer**. Again and again we are shown, how herbs are effective in disease prevention as well as cleansing the body of harmful substances. – Use the herbs and do your body a favour; it will keep you healthy and strong.

DIRECTIONS

Infusion: Mistletoe tea is made as a cold infusion. A heaped teaspoon of Mistletoe is soaked in ¼ litre of cold water overnight, the next morning slightly warmed and strained. If a larger amount per day is needed, the tea is kept in a thermos flask that has been rinsed with hot water, or warmed in a water bath each time.

Tincture: This is bought as a preparation.

Fresh juice: Fresh leaves and twigs are washed and, still wet, put into the juice extractor.

Ointment: The fresh berries of the Mistletoe are stirred into the cold lard (used for chilblains).

PLANTAIN, RIBWORT (Plantago lanceolata)

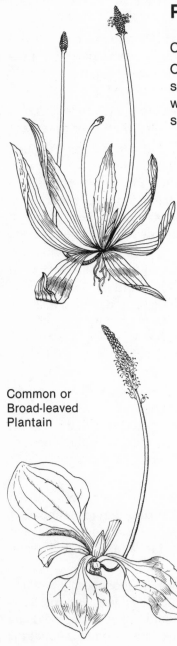

Common or Broad-leaved Plantain

Common names: Long Plantain, Ribble Grass, Snake Weed, Lamb's Tongue.

Of the many medicinal plants we know, this is one that has been as widespread and esteemed in ancient times as it is now. Since primeval times it was the ruler of the ways and grew for the benefit of mankind. An Anglo Saxon source mentions Plantain "Weybroed" as one of the nine sacred herbs:

"And you, Weybroed,
mother of plants,
open to the east
mighty inside:
Over you creak waggons,
over you rode women,
over you rode brides,
over you snorted horses.

You withstood all
and offered resistance.
So withstand too the venom
and contagion
and misfortune
that sweep across the land."

Today as then we need medicinal plants like Plantain which is so much esteemed in herbals. Its relative, the **Common Plantain** or Broad-leaved Plantain (Plantago major) has the same medicinal value and is used in the same way. Both grow by roadsides, in ditches, meadows, moist wastelands and may be found all over the world.

Primarily Plantain is used for all **disorders of the respiratory organs**, especially for **phlegm in the lungs, whooping cough, bronchial asthma**, even for **tuberculosis of the lungs**. The Swiss Abbé and herbalist Kuenzle, who knew much about the medicinal properties of herbs wrote: "The whole plant, roots, flowers and seeds of the Plantain is used. Like no other herb it cleanses the blood, the lungs and the stomach and is therefore valuable to those people who have little or **bad blood, weak lungs and kidneys, pale looks, eczema and herpes**, who are **hoarse and plagued with slight coughs** or who are as skinny as goats that not even wrapping them in butter would help. If **weak children**, despite good food, stay so, it helps them back on their feet."

I, myself, was able to help many a person suffering from **bronchial asthma**, with Thyme and Plantain used in equal proportions (see "directions"). Such an infusion is also recommended for **liver and bladder disorders**.

For **bronchitis, lung and bronchial asthma** the tea is made as follows. One cup of cold water, with a slice of lemon (without skin if sprayed) and 1 heaped teaspoon of raw sugar, is brought to the boil. When just off the boil, 1 teaspoon of the tea mixture is added and steeped for half a minute. For bad cases the tea is freshly prepared 4 to 5 times a day and taken in sips as hot as possible.

In old herbals you can read that the seeds are used for the prevention of **stones** if you eat 8 gm. daily and drink Chicory tea. Plantain syrup rids the blood of toxins and you should take 1 tablespoon (children 1 teaspoonful) before each meal for 3 weeks (see "directions").

Farmers know that Plantain is an old esteemed **remedy for wounds**. One day I watched a farmer, who had injured himself in the field, pick Plantain leaves, crush them and place them on the wound. Despite the unwashed leaves there was no infection. The fresh, bruised leaves are applied on **cuts, scratches, stings from poisonous insects, dog bites and snake bites**. For the latter it is a stopgap measure if no doctor is nearby. An old herbal states: "If the toad is bitten by a spider, it hurries to the Plantain to get help."

For **goitre** the fresh leaves are crushed between the hands, mixed with a bit of salt and applied to the throat. To keep the feet free from **blisters** on long walks, some leaves are put in the shoes. Even **malignant growths** disappear if treated with fresh, crushed leaves. They are also benificial for **malignant glandular disorders**. In this case it is also good to macerate fresh Marjoram (in urgent cases, dried Marjoram will do) in olive oil. The Marjoram is put in a bottle, oil is poured over it and it is left in a warm place for 10 days. The Marjoram oil so derived is brushed on the affected glands, the crushed Plantain leaves are placed over it and bandaged with a cloth. Soon an improvement is noted.

During one of my talks I said that the crushed leaves of Plantain would heal every **wound**, be it 10 years old. 5 month later, in another talk in the same town, a woman stated; "I was very sceptical about Plantain healing even old wounds. I have a neighbour who had **open sores** on her foot for 17 years and was therefore unable to go outside her house. I took Plantain leaves to her and applied them according to your directions on the sore foot. I had to retract my doubts. To everyone's surprise the wound soon healed and in the past 5 months has not re-opened."

Another example: An ex-serviceman with an artificial leg had **open sores on the stump** caused by the long summer heat. These would not heal; no ointment, injection or X-ray treatment gave relief. When he applied Plantain leaves the sores healed almost overnight and he could go back to work.

Years ago I was able to help myself with fresh Plantain juice. While carrying my then one year old grandchild in my arms, it suddenly bit into my left cheek above the corner of the mouth. For a few day this was quite painful. From time to time I dabbed the spot with Plantain herb essence. Suddenly one day I felt a pea-size hard lump where I had been bitten. Immediately I picked some Plantain leaves, crushed them between finger and thumb and dabbed the **lump** with it frequently during the day. In the evening, this lump was already softer and the next morning completely gone, to everyone's relief. It is not an exaggeration when the Abbé Kneipp says in his writings that there is a herb growing for every disease. The longer I deal with herbs, the more miracles I find. Many people die from malignant growths each year, althought there are plants for this. How much healthier and happier we would be, had we more understanding of our herbs which grow all around us. In many people's eyes they are only "weeds". Take the trouble to find out about herbs and your complaint will disappear gradually.

These lines of mine should also give hope to old people who suffer from **open sores** on legs for years. The sores will soon heal if Plantain leaves are used as a poultice. Age is of no importance. Should there also be a swelling, the foot is bathed first in a cold infusion of Mallow or a decoction of Horsetail. The edges of the sores are coated with Calendula ointment (see "directions Calendula"). Plantain leaves are also recommended for **thrombosis**.

These examples show clearly that one can still rely on God's pharmacy when a doctor's help is of no more avail.

DIRECTIONS

Infusion: One heaped teaspoon of leaves to ¼ litre of boiling water, infused for a short time.

Tea mixture: Equal proportions of Plantain and Thyme are mixed, 1 teaspoonful to ¼ litre of boiling water (see above text).

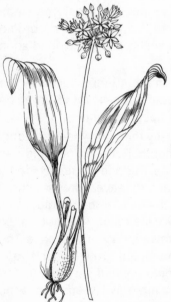

RAMSONS (Allium ursinum)

Common names: Wild Garlic, Broad-leaved Garlic, Wood Garlic, Bear's Garlic.

Every spring brings new hope and warmth. We feel joy and our thoughts have wings, we are pleased about the first sign of green, the singing of the birds and feel with our whole heart that all this is a gift of our Creator. In view of all this new splendour we should **cleanse our system and rid** it of **waste matters**.

The green, shiny broad leaves are very similar to those of the Lily-of-the-Valley. They grow from an elongated bulb, which is surrounded by layers of clear skin. The smooth, light-green stem, with its head of white flowers, grows to a height of 30 cm. Ramsons grows only in shady and damp woods. Its pungent garlic odour that has given it the name of Wild Garlic, is smelled long before the plants are sighted and prevents them from being mistaken for the Lilly-of-the-Valley or the Meadow Saffron (Colchicum autumnale).

In early spring many damp woods are densely carpeted with the fresh green leaves of Ramsons. They start to grow in April and May, sometimes earlier, the flowers from May to June. Powerful medicinal properties lie within Ramsons and it is related, that bears, after hibernation, seek it out to cleanse their system. Ramsons has similar medicinal properties to those of the Garlic, only greater. It is therefore especially valuable for a **"spring" course of treatment** to cleanse the system and to aid recovery from **chronic skin disorders**.

Since the leaves, when dried, loose their medicinal properties, they are used fresh for a spring cleaning and waste removal course of treatment. They are finely chopped and laid on buttered bread, used uncooked as a seasoning in the daily soup and added to potatoes, dumplings and other foods, where normally Parsley is used. The leaves can also be prepared like spinach or salad. Since they have a biting taste when used in large amounts, they should be mixed with Stinging Nettle leaves when prepared as a spinach dish.

The young leaves are gathered in April and May before the time of flowering, the bulbs in late summer and autumn. These bulbs can be used the same way as garlic. People who have a sensitive stomach should pour warm milk over the finely chopped leaves and bulbs, infuse them for two to three hours and sip this liquid.

To have the Ramsons' medicinal properties at home throughout the year, a Ramsons spirit is prepared (see "directions"). 10 to 12 drops of this are taken in water daily. These drops help to attain an excellent **memory**, prevent **arteriosclerosis** and dispel many other complaints.

Ramsons is beneficial for the stomach and intestines. It is most suitable for **acute and chronic diarrhoea** even when this is associated with **flatulence and colic**, as well as for **constipation** when this is caused by inactivity or sluggishness of the intestines. **Worms**, even **maw-worms** are expelled some time after eating Ramsons. Those complaints which occur in elderly or over-indulgent people, through sluggish or over-filled intestines, vanish with the improved intestinal activity. **Heart complaint and sleeplessness** arising from stomach trouble and those complaints, caused by **arteriosclerosis or high blood pressure**, as well as **dizziness, pressure in the head and anxiety**, diminish. The pressure decreases gradually. Ramsons' wine (see "directions") is a wonderful remedy for all old people with persisting **phlegm** in the chest and the connected **shortness of breath**. This remedy is also recommended for **consumption and dropsy**, from which old people often suffer. Leaves, used fresh, cleanse kidneys and bladder and increase the flow of urine. **Badly healing wounds**, brushed with the fresh juice, heal quickly. Even **disorders of the coronary blood vessels** can be relieved.

Ramsons, that has proved itself as a **blood-cleanser** for skin disorders, is not valued highly enough. The Swiss herbalist, Abbé Kuenzle especially praises the plant: "It cleanses the whole body, rids it of stubborn waste matters, produces healthy blood and destroys and removes poisonous substances. Continually sickly people, as those with **herpes** and eczema, pale looks, **scrofula and rheumatism**, should venerate Ramsons like gold. No herb on this earth is as effective for cleansing the stomach, intestines and blood. Young people would burst into bloom like the roses on a trellis and sprout like fir-cones in the sun." Kuenzle states further he knew families that, previously sickly, seeking remedy the whole year, covered in rashes, herpes, scrofula and pale faced, as if they had lain in the grave and been scratched out by the hens, became completely healthy and refreshed after long applications of this wonderful gift of God.

DIRECTIONS

Seasoning: Fresh leaves, finely chopped like chives or parsley, are sprinkled on bread, in soups, sauces, salads and meat dishes.

Ramsons' spirit: A bottle is loosely filled to the neck with finely chopped leaves or bulbs, which are covered with 38 % to 40 % rye whisky or other grain alcohol and placed in the sun or near the stove for 14 days. 10 to 15 drops are taken in water 4 times daily.

Ramsons' wine: A handful of finely chopped leaves is boiled for a short time in approx. ¼ litre of white wine, sweetened to taste with honey or syrup and sipped slowly.

SAGE (Salvia officinalis)

Common names: Garden Sage and Common Sage. – Sage, the familiar plant of the kitchen garden, comes to us from southern Europe. It grows to a height of 70 cm. and its purplish flowers are set in whorls. The leaves set in pairs on the stem are greyish-green with a silvery sheen and wrinkled. They possess a somewhat bitter, aromatic scent. Sage should grow in a sunny but sheltered position in your garden. To protect it from the frost, I cover it with branches of fir.

Another kind, the **Meadow Sage** (Salvia pratensis) grows on banks, in meadows and pastures. The showy, purplish-blue flowers exude an aromatic perfume and are used mainly as a **gargle** or to make **Sage vinegar** – a handful of flowers are macerated in natural vinegar – and this is used as a beneficial and invigorating rub or massage during long illnesses. The leaves are gathered before the flowers open and at midday in bright sunshine, since the volatile oils of the plant are only fully developed in sunshine. The leaves are dried in the shade.

It is about the Common or Garden Sage, whose medicinal properties are more powerful, that I would like to talk. Already among our forefathers it was a highly esteemed herb. A thirteenth century verse says:

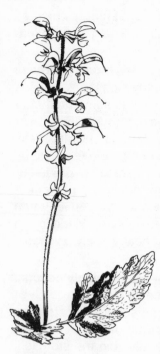

"Why should a man die, whilst Sage grows in his garden?" Sage is well named, coming from the Latin "salvare", to save, in reference to its curative properties.

How highly it was praised in olden times we can read in a delightful old herbal: "During the Virgin Mary's flight from Herod, all flowers in the field were asked to hide Her and the Baby Jesus, but none gave her shelter except Sage. After Herod's men had gone without seeing Her and the danger had passed, the Virgin Mary told the Sage: "From now to eternity, you will be the favourite flower of mankind. I give you the power to heal man of all illness and save him from death as you have done for me." Since then Sage grows to the benefit of mankind.

Sage tea, drunk frequently, strengthens the body, prevents **stroke** and is good for **paralysis**. Sage, besides Lavender, is the only plant that will help relieve **night sweats**; it attacks the illness which is the cause of it, and its invigorating forces take away the great weakness that is part of it. Many physicians have realized the beneficial qualities of Sage; they use it with great success for **cramps, disorders of the spinal cord, glandular disorders and for trembling of the limbs.** For these disorders 2 cups are sipped throughout the day. This tea is valuable in **liver** complaints, dispels **flatulence** and all complaints caused by an ill liver. It is blood **cleansing**, dispels **phlegm from the respiratory organs** and the **stomach**, increases the **appetite**, rectifies **intestinal trouble and diarrhoea.**

For **insect stings** crushed leaves are applied.

Sage tea is used for **ulcerated throat and mouth, inflammation of the tooth pulp, tonsillitis and throat disorders.** Many children and grown-ups could have saved themselves a tonsillectomy had they taken Sage tea in time. When the tonsils, which are the policemen of the body for toxic substances, are missing, the toxic substances go directly to the kidneys. A decoction of Sage is a useful gargle for **loose and bleeding teeth and ulcerated or receding gums.** A small piece of cotton saturated with Sage tea can be applied.

A sitz bath (see "directions") taken once in a while would be of great help to women with **abdominal troubles** and to people with **weak nerves.**

Besides its medicinal properties Sage is used as a culinary herb. In small quantities similar to Thyme and Savory it is added to pork, goose and turkey, not only for the aroma but also for breaking down the fat in the meat. A small leaf added to venison improves the taste. In some districts "Sage biscuits" are baked. Finely shredded leaves are added to the dough. Sage added to the cheese or sauces makes them wholesome.

DIRECTIONS

Infusion: ¼ litre of boiling water is poured over 1 teaspoon of herbs, infused for a short time.

Sage vinegar: A bottle is filled loosely to the neck with the flowers of the Meadow Sage, natural vinegar is poured over them, so that the flowers are covered and kept in a warm or sunny place for 14 days.

Sitz bath: Two heaped double handfuls of leaves are steeped in cold water overnight. Next day it is brought to the boil and the liquid is added to the bath water. (see General Information "sitz bath").

SHEPHERD'S PURSE (Capsella bursa-pastoris)

Common names: Mother's Heart, Pickpurse, Pickpocket, Lady's Purse and Rattle Pouches.

This herb is to be found everywhere in meadows, ditches, fields and gardens and is looked upon as a troublesome weed. Hardly any earth is moved — especially when building a house — without Shepherd's Purse growing almost overnight.

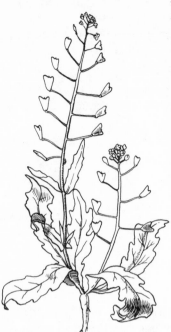

The irregular toothed lower leaves form a rosette — similar to Dandelion. The stems grow to a height of 40 cm. It flowers from spring through to autumn. The tiny, dirty-white flowers are borne in terminal clusters, the lower ones already succeeded by seed vessels, in the form of little heart-shaped pouches that feel leathery to the touch. Chickens have a special liking for these little pouches. As soon as the snow melts and nature is free from frost, the Shepherd's Purse grows fresh and green again.

Shepherd's Purse tea, 2 to 3 cups daily, is used with great success for all **kinds of bleedings**, as for example, **nose, stomach, intestinal and uterine bleeding**. A decoction of Shepherd's Purse is most effective for **wounds** which will not stop bleeding.

2 cups (1 heaped teaspoon per cup) are drunk daily, 8 to 10 days before the onset of menstruation, in cases of **excessive menstrual flow**. This tea also helps to regulate menstruation during **puberty**. During **menopause** every woman should drink 2 cups daily for 4 weeks, suspend the treatment for 3 weeks and then repeat the cycle.

For bleeding **haemorrhoids**, small enemas are given; washings and sitz baths with a luke warm decoction of Shepherd's Purse are taken. Nursing mothers with **swollen breasts** should steam the fresh Shepherd's Purse in a sieve and apply warm between cloths. 2 cups daily, of equal proportions of Horsetail and Shepherd's Purse, are recommended as a tea for bleeding from the **kidneys**.

The Shepherd's Purse — similar to the Mistletoe — is a circulation equalizing herb, recommended for **high** as well as for **low blood pressure**. Contrary to Mistletoe which must be prepared cold, this tea is infused with boiling water. Two cups are taken daily and stopped when the circulation has become normal. Like Mistletoe, Shepherd's Purse is good for **uterine bleeding**. The tea in this case is drunk only for some time.

For all **external muscular disorders** this valuable medicinal herb is an especially important aid. It is interesting that nothing is found about it in almost all new herbals. A few years ago, an elderly man gave me a beautiful, old herbal with unique prints and drawings. As it goes, when the day is filled from morning to late evening, I was unable to look through it. One day towards midnight I suddenly awoke, as if I were being gently shaken by the shoulders. The thought came to me: "Now you have had the herbal for six months and have not read through it once." I arose wide awake, got the book and sat comfortably in the living room. I opened it and immediately a few lines jumped to my eyes: "For **limb or muscular atrophy** if nothing else helps take this: Shepherd's Purse, finely chopped, macerated in Rye spirits and kept in the sun or near the stove for 10 days, then rubbed well into the skin several times daily; 4 cups of Lady's Mantle tea are taken internally." As if it were intended I should read these few lines — in that moment I was not aware of it — I closed the book, put it in its place, went back to bed and was asleep in a short time. A few days later I received a telephone call from Vienna: "Could you help me. I am 52 years old, a nurse and for 2 years in early retirement. I am completely helpless with **muscular atrophy**." When I had given her the above recipe and when she came 3 weeks later in good health to see me, I learned that on the day that I was awoken at midnight, she had made a pilgrimage to San Damiano in Italy. On the way back in the bus, a man who saw her affliction, referred her to me. A short time later she was sufficiently strengthened to take up nursing again.

Another call, this time from Upper Austria: "I am 62 years old. Because of a **weak anus muscle** I had a **prolapse of the rectum** which was operated on. This autumn the same thing happened again. Day and night I suffered continous pain from the navel to the hips. The doctors in the hospital declined a second operation, there was nothing more to do." I immediately thought of Shepherd's Purse and recommended 4 cups of Lady's Mantle tea daily which strengthens the internal muscle and externally, a Shepherd's Purse tincture, used as a rub or massage, and 10 drops of which are added 3 times a day to the tea. During the 10 days that are needed to prepare the tincture, I recommended the use of Swedish Bitters compresses. My surprise was unimaginable, when the woman rang me after a time to tell me all her complaints had gone. The prolapsed rectum was corrected, the anus muscle functioned normally and the terrible pain in the hips had already eased 2 days after the start of the treatment. One can only say: How the medicinal herbs of God's Pharmacy help! Who makes such miracles happen? Only the grace of the Creator!

A woman from Lower Austria wrote: "During a lecture I asked you about **hernia**. While the Shepherd's Purse tincture was macerating, I applied compresses of Swedish Bitters. Then I started to massage with Shepherd's Purse tincture and drank 4 cups of Lady's Mantle tea daily. I did this for 6 weeks. Since, as a farmer's wife, I could not take it easy — it was harvest time — I wore a support. After 12 days of treatment there was no sign of the hernia, although I still felt pain. 2 months later, it too was gone."

The since deceased medical superintendent Dr. Erich Roehling of the sanatorium near Garmisch, Bavaria, who had visited me once, read this letter and was visibly impressed. He thought that from a medical point of view hernia could only be corrected by an operation.

Internally 4 cups of Lady's Mantle tea, and Shepherd's Purse tincture used externally as a rub or massage are also effective for **prolapse of the uterus** (the massage is done from the genitals up to the abdomen). I want to emphasize that the tincture has to be prepared from freshly picked Shepherd's Purse. For such serious muscular disorders only fresh herbs give swift and sure relief!

DIRECTIONS

Infusion: 1 heaped teaspoon per ¼ litre of boiling water, infused for a short time.

Sitz bath: See General Information "sitz bath".

Compress: 1 heaped double handful of Shepherd's Purse, if possible the fresh herb, is placed in a sieve over boiling water. The moist, warm herb is put between a cloth and applied.

Tincture: Freshly picked Shepherd's Purse, the leaves, stems, flowers and seed pods are finely cut and placed loosely into a bottle to the neck, 38% to 40% rye whisky is poured over it (the herbs have to be covered) and left in the sun or in a warm place for 10 days.

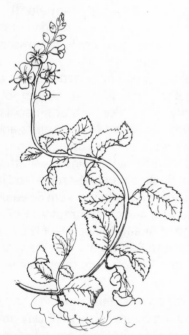

SPEEDWELL (Veronica officinalis)

Common names are Veronica, Bird's Eye, Ground-well and Common Speedwell.

When the Romans conquered Germanic lands, they learned from the old Teutons about the great value of this much esteemed herb. The Romans, as I read in an old herbal, must have been convinced of this herb's great value. If they wanted to compliment an acquaintance of a friend, they said he had as many good qualities as the highly esteemed Speedwell.

This saying I remembered, when one day a gentleman told me of the high **cholesterol level** in his blood. He had been to hospital several times. I recommended Speedwell, two cups per day. My pleasure was great when, six months later he told me the doctors were surprised there was no high level of cholesterol, when shortly ago they gave him a check-up.

Speedwell likes dry ground and grows in woods, copses, heaths, hedgerows, edges of woodlands and paths. It has a creeping, hairy stem with little finely-toothed silvery leaves and clusters of light-blue to purplish flowers. When touched the leaves fall off easily. The time of flowering is May to August. The flowerheads are gathered. Most effective are those plants which grow on the edge of woods and under oaks.

This traditional herb is a favourite addition to teas that **cleanse the blood** and, together with fresh Stinging Nettle tops, it heals chronic **eczema**. It is especially recommended for **senile pruritis**. Weak people tolerate it as a **stomachic** of gentle action which also stimulates digestion. Fluids and mucus in the stomach and **intestinal disorders** are eliminated.

Speedwell is efficacious for old, dry **bronchitis**. For chest complaints, a tea is made from an equal proportions mixture of Lungwort (Pulmonaria officinalis), Coltsfoot, Plantain and Speedwell, sweetened with honey or raw sugar.

I would like to point out that Speedwell has a great medicinal value for **nervousness** caused by **mental over exertion**. One cup drunk before going to bed, through its soothing effect, is highly beneficial. The Abbé Kuenzle recommends this soothing tea to people who have to work a lot with their head. It brings **good memory** and disperses **dizziness**. Mixed with Celery roots it rectifies **weak nerves** as well as **depression**. Even for **jaundice and gravel** in the **bladder, rheumatic and gout** pain in the limbs, Speedwell is very effective.

A priest relates: "My **memory lapses** disappeared surprisingly after drinking tea, prepared of equal amounts of Speedwell and Horsetail (2 cups per day). I had become uncertain and worried, when during sermons I forgot important words. The herbs have helped very quickly."

For **jaundice, liver and spleen disorders**, I recommend the following mixture; 50 gm. Dandelion roots, 25 gm. Wild Chicory flowers (Cichorium intybus), 25 gm. Woodruff (Asperula odorata) and 50 gm. Speedwell. 2 cups of this unsweetened tea are sipped throughout the day (1 heaped teaspoon of herbs per cup of boiling water).

The fresh juice prepared from the flowering plant, is recommended for **chronic skin disorders**, especially for **eczema** (see "directions"). One teaspoonful of the juice is taken 3 times a day. I recommend Speedwell, in old herbals praised as a wound-herb, for all **inflamed, non-healing wounds**, especially wounds near the shinbone. The wound is washed with a decoction of Speedwell and then compresses made from the freshly prepared infusion are applied, wrapped up warmly and left on overnight.

People who suffer from **rheumatism and gout** should try the easily prepared Speedwell tincture (see "directions"). This tincture is used externally as a friction; internally 15 drops in water or tea are taken three times a day.

Be sure to drink a tea prepared from the freshly picked herb for a period every year! Speedwell not only prevents **arteriosclerosis**, it gives the body new elasticity through its **purifying action**. Therefore my request: Take my advice!

DIRECTIONS

Infusion: 1 heaped teaspoon of herbs per cup of boiling water, infused for a short time.

Fresh juice: The freshly picked flower heads are washed and, still wet, put into the juice extractor. The juice is poured into small bottles and stored in the refrigerator.

Tincture: 1 heaped double handful of the finely chopped flowering plant is macerated in 1 litre of 38% rye whisky or wodka and placed in the sun or near the stove for 14 days.

Tea mixture: 1 heaped teaspoon per cup of boiling water, infused for a short time.

STINGING NETTLE (Urtica dioica)

In a radio program a physician once pointed out that the Stinging Nettle is one of our most valuable medicinal herbs. Mankind does not realize how valuable it is or it would plant Stinging Nettles (common name is Greater Nettle) only.

Everything of the Nettle, stems, leaves, flowers and roots, has medicinal properties. In ancient times it was already highly esteemed. Albrecht Duerer (1471 – 1528) painted an angel who flies heavenwards with Stinging Nettles in his hands. The Swiss herbalist Abbé Kuenzle points out in his writings that the Nettle would have been wiped out long ago were it not for its stings. Insects and animals would have eaten it away.

I once told a mother of 7 children who since the last birth had suffered from **eczema and headaches**, to drink Nettle tea. In a short time she was free from the eczema and the headaches too. Since the cause of eczema often lies internally, it has to be treated internally with blood cleansing herbs. Stinging Nettle is our best **blood cleansing and blood building** herb. Since it has a good influence over the pancreas, it assists in lowering the **blood sugar**. It remedies **disorders and inflammation of the urinary passage and supression of urine**. It stimulates the **movements of the bowel** and is therefore recommended as a spring course of treatment.

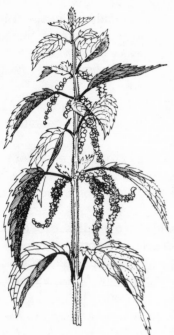

Since I know how valuable the Nettle is, I have made it a habit to drink a tea prepared from the young shoots during a 4 week period each spring and autumn. I drink 1 cup on an empty stomach half an hour before breakfast and sip 1 to 2 cups throughout the day. The effect is heightened if the tea is only sipped, even before breakfast. After 4 weeks, I feel like a new person and I am able to work 3 times as hard. My family and I have not taken any medication for years and I feel young and supple. The Stinging Nettle tea is drunk without sugar and does not taste too badly. Delicate natures can add a bit of Camomile or Mint to better the taste. In herbal medicine Stinging Nettle tea drunk during a 4 week period, is used for **liver, gallbladder and spleen disorders**, even for a **tumour in the spleen, for stomach cramps and ulcers, ulcers in the intestines, congestion of the lungs or stomach and lung disorders**. Do not boil the tea, it would destroy valuable substances. Drink 1 cup a day all year round as a prophylactic. It is also beneficial for **viral diseases and bacterial excretions**.

From a certain age on the body has less iron and there are symptoms of **fatigue and exhaustion**; one feels old and less efficient. The Stinging Nettle with its **iron content** is used with great success and after a period energy, vitality and a bodily well-being is experienced.

A young, an(a)emic looking woman once came to see me. She suffered from stomach and gall bladder disorders and as a side effect from **head-aches**. I recommended Stinging Nettle tea. Some time later I met her by chance and excitedly she told me how quickly Stinging Nettle tea had helped her. Her whole family has turned to herbs.

Stinging Nettle is diuretic and therefore of value for **dropsy**. As a blood builder it is beneficial for **anaemia, chlorosis** and other **blood disorders**. Together with other herbs the Stinging Nettle is successfully employed in **leukaemia** (see article on leukaemia, page 79). People who suffer from **allergies** (including **hay fever**) should drink Stinging Nettle tea for a while.

The Stinging Nettle diminishes **susceptibility to colds** and helps in cases of **gout and rheumatism**. A lady who suffered from **sciatica** was under medical care for 3 years. After 6 Stinging Nettle baths (200 gm. of Nettles per bath) she lost all pain within 6 months.

I met a woman, about 50 years old, who had such **thin hair** that she had to wear a wig which would have caused the rest of the hair to fall out, too. I recommended a Stinging Nettle tea hair wash, made from a mixture of Stinging Nettle tea and a decoction of Stinging Nettle roots. She took my advice and from week to week her hair improved and grew much thicker. Very beneficial for hair is the Stinging Nettle tincture, easily prepared from the roots dug up in spring or autumn (see "directions"). I, myself, rub this tincture into the scalp daily; even on trips I take it with me. It is worth the effort, no dandruff, the hair is thick and soft and has a beautiful sheen.

For **vascular constrictions** (Buerger's disease) Stinging Nettle is most beneficial. Many a person could have saved himself an amputation of the leg by taking Stinging Nettle foot baths in time (see "directions").

Every cramp, no matter where, means a **faulty circulation**. Washing and bathing with a decoction of Stinging Nettle is recommended. For **coronary artery constriction** it is also recommended. Bend the chest over the bath tub and bathe the heart region together with a gentle massage with the luke warm tea.

A 51 year old woman from Bavaria had a **fistula** which caused her considerable pain for 28 years. An operation was questionable, since the fistula was on the cheekbone. In 1978, she went to see a nonmedical practitioner who put her on a fresh vegetable and fruit diet, prescribed deep and proper breathing and psychocybernetics; above everything he gave her sympathy. The pain became bearable, but the fistula was still there. In March, 1979, she started to gather the first young Nettles and to drink 3 cups of tea with 1 teaspoon of Swedish Bitters added to each cup daily. She wrote: "After exactly 2 weeks the fistula had disappeared and I was without pain. And it has stayed this way."

With pleasure I hear, again and again, that people have experienced the curative effect of Stinging Nettle. Not long ago, a woman wrote that she had drunk Nettle tea for months. Not only had she lost all fatigue and exhaustion, despite hard daily work, but also a festering **corn** which had caused her pain up to the thigh, as well as a **fungus under the nails**, had disappeared. Another woman wrote that finally she got rid of a painful **eczema**. Such letters are rays of hope in my life. They show that our medicinal herbs help whenever they are used.

An elderly man came to see me. 3 years ago he had influenza. Since that time his urine was dark brown and he suffered from terrible **headaches**. Neither the prescribed medications he took, nor the injections (lately in the head) brought relief. On the contrary, the headaches became worse; he was close to committing suicide. I gave him hope and recommended the Stinging Nettle. He was to drink 2½ litres of the tea throughout the day. After 4 days he rang up to say that he felt better than even before the influenza. Use the young Nettle tops, especially in spring, as a course of treatment. You will be surprised of its effects.

From a letter I quote: "Many thanks for your invaluable help. For 19 years I have been suffering and no physician could tell me what was wrong with me, although I consulted many. One week long I drank Nettle tea and miraculousy my illness was gone, as if I never had suffered." From these accounts it can be seen how quickly the herbs bring relief. Of course, 1 cup a day won't help, especially for bad cases at least 2 litres a day have to be sipped.

A business woman told me that she takes a thermos flask of Stinging Nettle tea on all her trips. She swears by it. It not only quenches the thirst but refreshes and takes away **weariness**.

A special hint: For **sciatica, lumbago and neuritis** in arms and legs, the affected parts are lightly brushed with a freshly picked Stinging Nettle. For sciatica, the Stinging Nettle is brushed upward from the foot along the outside to the hip and then downward on the inside towards the foot; repeated twice and then from the hips across the bottom. Similarly it is used for other affected areas. Afterwards the affected skin areas are powdered.

Don't we have to thank God for such wonderful herbs? In our fast living time man walks past them and prefers to use analgesics which he takes in excess.

I would like to tell of another experience which has touched me deeply. In our small town I met an elderly woman who suffered, as the doctor had diagnosed, from **cancerous growths in her stomach**. She could not decide to have an operation, because of her age. Someone told her to drink Stinging Nettle tea. So, every day, she went into her garden to pick a handful of Stinging Nettles from along the fence, where they grew in abundance. When, after a time, she went to see her doctor, he asked in surprise: "What happened?" The growths had disappeared and the woman could enjoy a healthy old age. There is no need to let it get that far. Never could a **malignant growth** form, if we not only valued the Stinging Nettle, but drank it as a tea in regular intervals.

Another good advice: Start today with a Stinging Nettle course of treatment. The dried herb can be bought at a herbal chemist. The Stinging Nettle, growing wild, can be picked in spring. The more freshly picked it is used, the greater are its medicinal properties. For the winter supply the Stinging Nettles gathered in May are best. Be pleased to be able to do something positive for your health!

A reader from Germany wrote: "My neighbour uses the Stinging Nettle to eradicate pests in his garden. He puts a large amount of Stinging Nettle in a container which holds approximate 300 litres (a smaller container can be used) and leaves them to soak for a while. With this Stinging Nettle water he sprays the plants again and again. He therefore grows plants free from pests without having to use chemicals."

Some farmers spray the Stinging Nettles, which grow on forest fringes and near paths away from roads and other pollutants, with herbicides. They do not consider that at the same time birds and valuable insects are killed. Many farmers do not take the time anymore to mow the Stinging Nettle with a scythe. How blind have we become!

DIRECTIONS

Infusion: 1 heaped teaspoon per ¼ litre of boiling water, infused for a short time.

Tincture: The roots, dug up in spring or autumn, are cleaned with a brush, chopped and placed in a bottle up to the neck. 38% to 40% rye whisky or wodka is poured over it and the bottle is left to stand in a warm place for 14 days.

Foot bath: 1 heaped handful of well washed roots and 1 heaped double handful of Stinging Nettle (stems and leaves) are soaked in 5 litres of cold water overnight. The next day this is brought to the boil and used 2 or 3 times.

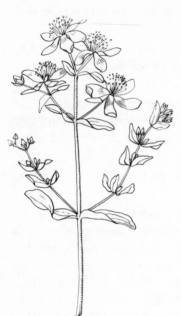

ST. JOHN'S WORT (Hypericum perforatum)

This plant grows in meadows, hedges, woodlands and on roadsides. It reaches a height of 60 cm., is much branched and its golden-yellow flowers, grouped in umbels, are easily recognized by the red juice they yield, when pressed between the fingers. The flowering plant is gathered for infusions and baths, the just opened flowers for the preparation of St. John's Wort oil.

Old Christian beliefs connected the fragrant, red juice of the flowers with the blood and wounds of Jesus Christ. The fact is that St. John's Wort oil is the best wound oil, it soothes the pain, is anti-inflammatory and healing. Legends dedicate this herb to Saint John the Baptist.

In earlier times, maidens twisted garlands of St. John's Wort and wore them, dancing around the fires on Saint John's day. In this mysterious night, branches of the herb were thrown into the water to show the maidens who would be their suitor in the next year.

According to an old custom, the farmers in Upper Austria fed St. John's Wort, placed between 2 layers of bread, to the animals to keep them free from all diseases. In these days it is done only rarely.

St. John's Wort tea is used for **injured nerves and nervous affections, for injuries** caused by a **blow** as well as a **consequence of strain**.

For **trigeminal neuralgia**, two to three cups of St. John's Wort tea are sipped daily and the affected area is rubbed with St. John's Wort oil. A tincture of St. John's Wort, easily prepared, is described as "Arnica of the nerves" and is effectively used for **nervous complaints, neuritis, neurosis, sleeplessness and nervous debility**.

Speech disorders, fitful sleep, hysterics, sleep walking are remedied with St. John's Wort, as well as **bed wetting and depressions**. My experiences show that for all these disorders, besides the use of the tea internally, sitz baths can be very beneficial (see "directions"). 1 sitz bath a week, followed by 6 consecutive foot baths. This course of treatment is recommended for all nervous complaints.

Girls during puberty should drink 2 cups of this tea daily for a length of time. It strengthens the female organs and promotes **regular menstruation**.

A much valued natural remedy is St. John's Wort oil. No home should be without it. It is easily prepared (see "directions") and keeps its healing properties for two years. It is not only used for **open wounds**, fresh wounds, **contusions and glandular swellings** and as an effective massage oil, it relieves **sore backs, lumbago, sciatica and rheumatism**. To have an effective remedy for **burns and scalds**, the flowers are macerated in linseed oil. This oil is also used for **sunburn**.

Babies, suffering from **abdominal pain**, are easily soothed by gently rubbing their tummy with St. John's Wort oil. I know a farmer's wife who uses this oil for all **injuries**, even on the animals. Her husband once hurt his hand badly in a machine. Compresses made of St. John's Wort soon eased the pain and the wound healed without problem. Another farmer treated his horse's external foot-injury with this oil.

A doctor diagnosed a **swelling of the lymphatic gland** in the abdomen of an 8 year old girl. Every time she was affected by the cold, internally or externally, she suffered from abdominal pain, especially in the morning. Her mother read that St. John's Wort oil is used successfully for all glandular swellings. Therefore she rubbed the child's stomach with this oil, every time she complained of pain, with success.

THYME, WILD THYME (Thymus serpyllum)

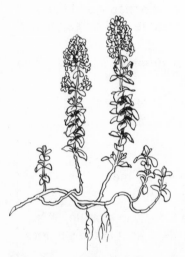

It grows on sundrenched rocky ground, in heaths, in dried-up lawns and near ant-hills. As it must have heat, it flourishes especially where the reflected heat from stones can reach it.

In the midday sun the dense purplish flower cushions perfume the air which attracts insects and bees to them. As long as I can remember these wonderful flowers with their aromatic fragrance have had a great attraction for me.

Thyme came to us from the Mediterranean countries during the eleventh century and the cultivated form, grown mainly in our gardens, is known as **Garden Thyme** (Thymus vulgaris) sometimes as Mother Thyme. Is grows taller than the Wild Thyme, up to 50 cm. Both plants have the same medicinal properties.

Thyme was well known in ancient times and old records state: "Thyme is most of all pungent and hot. It **increases the flow of urine and menstruation**, in normal birth speeds up delivery and dispatches **miscarriages** as well. A draught of it cleanses the noble internal parts of the body."

The Abbess Hildegard von Bingen refers to Thyme as a medicine for **leprosy, paralysis and nervous complaints**. He who drinks a cup of Thyme tea instead of coffee in the morning will soon feel the beneficial effect: enlivened spirits, great comfort in the stomach, no coughing in the morning and an overall well-being.

For **facial neuralgia** a herb pillow, made of Camomile, Thyme and Yarrow, picked in the sun and dried, is placed on the affected area and 2 cups of Thyme tea are sipped throughout the day. Should there be cramps, a Club Moss pillow is used as well.

A 79 year old farmer who had suffered from **facial neuralgia** for 27 years, had had a couple of operations, but it got worse. In the last couple of months, his mouth was pulled almost up to the ear and this caused great pain. First he used Swedish Bitters employed as a compress which brought a slight relief. Only after he used the above mentioned herb pillow did he benefit greatly from it. He kept drinking Thyme tea long after the neuralgia was gone.

My child, when 4 years old, after **typhoid fever**, could not regain its strength. For 2 years, we tried several things without success. Then, after a single Thyme bath lasting 20 minutes, a "different" child emerged. From this day on he simply blossomed.

Thyme is gathered during the time of flowering, from June to the beginning of autumn. Picked in the midday sun it is most effective. Thyme oil (see "directions") is used for **paralysis, stroke, multiple sclerosis, muscular atrophy, rheumatism and sprains**.

For **stomach and menstrual pain** as well as **abdominal cramps**, Thyme is recommended for internal and external use. Externally, Thyme picked in the sun and dried is applied as a herb pillow. Before going to sleep, the herb pillow is warmed in a pan and applied to the stomach or abdomen. This pillow is also recommended for **swellings and contusions**.

An old herbal remedy for **illnesses of the respiratory passages** is Thyme used with Plantain. A tea, made of equal proportions of Thyme and Plantain with lemon and raw sugar added, is effective for **whooping cough, phlegm in the lungs and bronchial asthma**. This tea is prepared fresh 4 to 5 times a day. If there is danger of **pneumonia**, a big sip, taken every hour, is effective. Luckily, many mothers have not forgotten Thyme, but seldom do they realize that drinks directly from the refrigerator can lead in children to **chronic bronchitis** which in later years can develop into **emphysema**.

Thyme tincture (see "directions") is used as a rub or massage to **strengthen the limbs** of weakly children; people who suffer from **multiple sclerosis** should use it, too.

A family could be spared a lot of trouble, if the sick child is treated in time with Thyme tea or Thyme baths. Many a nervous child has found a restful sleep after a Thyme bath. People who suffer from nervous **overstimulation or depressions** will find relief in a short time through such baths.

That Thyme is a recommended remedy for **alcoholism** should not be forgotten. Over a large handful of Thyme 1 litre of boiling water is poured, covered, infused for 2 minutes and poured into a thermos flask. The alcoholic is given a tablespoon of this tea every quarter of an hour. This results in nausea, vomiting, increased bowel action, increased flow of urine and perspiration, but also great appetite and thirst. In cases of relapses, which are inevitable in the beginning but later occur less and less, the treatment is repeated.

Thyme is also recommended for **epileptic fits**. The tea, 2 cups daily, should be drunk for a period of two to three weeks, with a 10 day interval, all year round.

Thyme syrup is tasty and digestible and, taken before meals, recommended for **colds**.

DIRECTIONS

Infusion: 1 heaped teaspoon per cup of boiling water, infused for a short time.

Bath: 200 gm. of Thyme for a full bath (see General Information "bath").

Tincture: The flowering herbs, picked in the midday sun, are placed loosely in a bottle, 38% to 40% rye whisky or wodka poured over them and the bottle is kept in the sun for fourteen days.

Thyme oil: The flowering herbs, picked in the midday sun, are placed loosely into a bottle. Cold pressed olive oil is poured over them to about 3 cm. above the plants. The bottle is left to stand in the sun or in a warm place for 14 days.

Herb pillow: The herbs are filled into a pillow and sown up.

Thyme syrup: In a pot, layers of moist Thyme, picked in the sun, and raw sugar are alternated and pressed down firmly. This is left in the sun for approx. 3 weeks; then strained and the residue rinsed in a small amount of water, strained again and added to the first liquid. This is heated gently on a low heat until the syrup is thick-flowing, testing the consistency from time to time.

WALNUT (Juglans regia)

Common names are Jupiter's Nut and Common Walnut. – The Walnut, a large tree, flowers in early spring, before the leaves appear. The leaves are gathered in June. The green, unripe fruit is gathered as long as a pin is easily inserted, the green husks are gathered before they turn brown and the nuts when ripe.

A tea of Walnut leaves **cleanses the blood** and is an effective remedy for **intestinal disorders**, as well as for **constipation and lack of appetite**. It is used successfully for **jaundice and diabetes**.

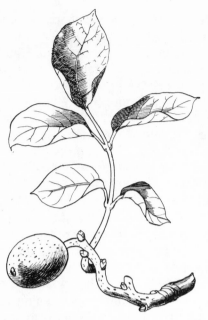

A decoction of the leaves, added to the bath water, is beneficial for **scrofula, rickets, caries and swellings of the bone**, as well as for **festering toe and finger nails**. An improvement is noted soon, if areas affected by **cradle-cap, scabs and scurf** are washed with a decoction of the green leaves.

Baths and washings enriched with this decoction are used for **acne, festering eczema, sweaty feet** and **leucorrhoea** ("whites"). As a mouthwash it is used for **stomatitis, inflamed gums, throat and larynx.**

A strong decoction of the leaves, added to the bath water is used for **chilblains**. It is also beneficial for **loss of hair**, when it is massaged frequently into the scalp. This decoction is also an excellent remedy for **headlice**. The fresh leaves are used to repel **insects**.

About the middle of June, the unripe nuts are picked (a pin should easily run through them) and used to prepare a delightful cordial, which cleanses **stomach, liver and blood**, strengthens **weak stomachs** and improves **foul intestines**. It is an excellent remedy for **thick blood**.

DIRECTIONS

Infusion: ¼ litre of boiling water is poured over 1 heaped teaspoon of finely cut leaves, infused for a short time.

Bath addition: 100 gm. of leaves per bath; for washings, 1 heaped teaspoon of cut leaves per cup of boiling water (see General Information "bath"). The double amount is used for a strong decoction.

Walnut cordial: Approx. 20 unripe nuts are quartered, put into a widenecked bottle and 1 litre of rye whisky is poured over them so that they are covered by 2 to 3 finger widths. Well stoppered, the bottle is kept in the sun or in a warm place for 2 to 4 weeks. The liquid is strained and bottled. According to need — 1 teaspoonful is taken. — A very palatable drink is obtained if 2 to 3 cloves, a piece of cinnamon stick, a small piece of vanilla pod, the washed, unsprayed rind of half an orange and 500 gm. of sugar, boiled in ¼ litre of water and cooled, are added to the strained cordial.

SMALL FLOWERED WILLOW-HERB (Epilobium parviflorum)

Once I received a letter from a family man in which it said, I quote: "I beg you to show me a way back to health and give my family back their healthy father." Before, he had related his story: In 1961 a chronic **inflammation of the prostate gland** became acute through bathing in water containing radium. He went from one hospital to another, no doctor operated on him, he was in despair. Every time he had a bowel movement, there was pus and blood in the stools. Due to the many medications he developed duodenal ulcers, serious liver disorders and the valuable intestinal bacteria were destroyed. He became very sick and, on the doctor's orders, had to stop all medication. Then he was, as he wrote, operated on electrically. Despite the operation the inflammation did not clear up. Medications and injections worsened his condition again. Then he started to drink Stinging Nettle tea and a special tea for bladder trouble, which improved his condition so far that he was able to go back to work. He could have spared himself all this suffering had he but known the Small Flowered Willow-herb which can cure disorders of the prostate gland.

The Willow-herb, until now hardly found mentioned in herbals, has since the first publication of this book in the German language started an almost triumphal march across Europe and even further, as a medicinal herb for disorders of the **prostate gland.**

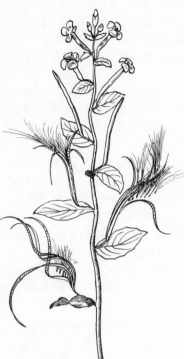

Since there are several species of Willow-herb and some people are uncertain which are the ones with the medicinal properties I will mention the ones that can be used: **Pink Willow-herb** (Epilobium roseum), **Small flowered Willow-herb** (Epilobium parviflorum), **Mountain Willow-herb** (Epilobium montanum), **Dark-green Willow-herb** (Epilobium obscurum), **Lance-leaved Willow-herb** (Epilobium lanzeolatum), **Hill Willow-herb** (Epilobium collinum), **Marsh Willow-herb** (Epilobium palustre), **Gravel Willow-herb** (Epilobium fleischeri), and **Alpine Willow-herb** (Epilobium anagallidifolium). The Willow-herbs with the medicinal properties are recognizable by their small flowers. The colour is reddish, pale-pink to almost white. The flowers stand on top of the long thin pod-like seed vessels. These later split, disclosing many silky white hairs in which are embedded the tiny seeds.

Of the varieties mentioned, the whole herb is gathered, that is, stems with leaves and flowers, but care should be taken to pick the herb in the middle of the stem — it breaks easily — so that it can form new side shoots. The plant is cut in the fresh state. Even in the most severe cases only 2 cups of Willow-herb tea are drunk, 1 cup in the morning on an empty stomach and 1 cup in the evening. But it does not mean that a visit to the doctor is not necessary. In any case, for every serious illness, a doctor has to be consulted.

2 species of Willow-herb which can hardly be mistaken for the smaller species are the **Great Hairy Willow-herb** (Epilobium hirsutum) and the **Rose Bay Willow-herb** (Epilobium angustifolium). These must not be gathered. The first has large rose-purple flowers. It grows, much branched, in masses by ponds, in marshes and damp meadows and reaches a height of 150 cm. The stems and leaves are fleshy and slightly hairy. The Austrian botanist, Richard Willfort, who knew the Willow-herb as a medicinal plant well, does not mention it in his book. As he said, it could be easily mistaken for the Great Hairy Willow-herb which, compared to the Small Flowered Willow-herb, has flowers 5 times as large, its stems and leaves are fleshy and it grows a lot taller, but has the opposite effect. The **Rose Bay Willow-herb** (Epilobium angustifolium) also know as Fireweed, Blood Vine, Blooming Sally, grows in copses, waste grounds recently cleared and edges of woods and reaches a height of 150 cm. The slightly reddish stems end in long showy spikes of rose-purple flowers. When these abundantly growing Rose Bay Willow-herbs flower, they turn areas into fire-red patches.

I was a young woman, when my father-in-law, in his prime, died from **hypertrophy of the prostate gland**. A neighbour who knew a lot about herbs showed me the Small Flowered Willow-herb and said: "Had your father-in-law drunk the tea made from this plant he would still be alive today. Take note of this plant! You are still a young woman and you might be able to help a lot of people." But as things go when one is young and healthy, I did not trouble myself about it. Not so my mother! She gathered Willow-herb every year and was able to help many people suffering from **bladder or kidney disorders**. The curative effect is so great that, often suddenly, all complaints caused by **prostate disorder** disappear. There were cases, where men were to have an operation, the urine came only in drops and 1 cup of this tea brought relief. Of course, the tea has to be drunk throughout a period to bring about complete recovery.

Through my mother I heard of a patient who had undergone 3 operations for clinically diagnosed **cancer of the bladder** and who was in a sad state. I recommended Willow-herb tea. Later I heard from his doctor that he had recovered. This happened at a time when I did not concern myself with medicinal herbs. But this case had a lasting effect on me. My mother often told me not to forget to gather Willow-herb should she be gone one day. In 1961 my dear mother died and I forgot to gather Willow-herb that summer. In the surgery of my doctor I learned that an acquaintance of mine was in hospital with cancer of the bladder. I thought of the Willow-herb. The doctor, although not against herbs, said that in this case nothing could help. But I had not gathered any Willow-herb and noticed with dismay that it was now the middle of October, everything would be wilted and dried up. Nevertheless I went to a place where I had seen them flowering in the summer. I found only some yellowed stems which I picked and cut finely. This I sent to the man's wife. She gave him 2 cups a day, 1 cup in the morning and 1 cup in the evening. 14 days later, the doctor rang me up to say that this man was feeling much better. "Well, your herbs help!", he said laughingly. From that time on I have been able to help hundreds and hundreds of people. As an old man once had said to me: "Take note of this plant! You might be able to help many people."

A chemist in Munich showed me an old pharmacopoeia where it was still mentioned around 1880. Drugs have pushed it aside. Through my publications, talks and herb-walks the Willow-herb has become known again. My suggestions find an echo in many people, thence when my husband and I go on our walks, be it in the mountains, on hills or near brooks, we meet with pleasure people picking out carefully the middle shoot of the Willow-herb. Everyone who knows this herb values and preserves it through careful picking. It grows back 2 or 3 times after being picked.

From many letters I learned that in many gardens the Willow-herb grows between strawberries, vegetables and flowers and for many years it was looked upon as a troublesome weed and pulled out. How it could have helped many a suffering person. Not so long ago I was able to help a priest who, suffering from **cancer of the prostate gland** and given up by the doctors, is now doing his normal work.

From a letter I quote: "My sister-in-law suffered from a tear in the intestine and the bladder caused by X-ray treatment. It was so painful that the doctor had to give her morphine. According as per the illustration in your book 'Health through God's Pharmacy', we looked for the Small Flowered Willow-herb, found it and gave the tea to my sister-in-law. After having drunk the tea for one week the pain subsided."

Many who suffer from a **disorder of the prostate gland** are able to find relief without an operation through the Willow-herb. If an operation has been performed, the Willow-herb tea relieves the burning and other complaints which often occur afterwards. But in any case a doctor should be consulted.

A man who had recovered from a **prostate disorder** wrote: "The Small Flowered Willow-herb has relieved my prostate disorder. I was in hospital with a heart infarct but I also suffered from prostate disorder and because of my heart trouble I could not be operated on. I heard of the wonderful Willow-herb which has helped in so many similar cases. I started to drink 3 cups daily; after several days I had no more complaints. I still drink 2 cups per day for a complete recovery. I thank God from the bottom of my heart. May you, Mrs. Treben, help many more people with the Small Flowered Willow-herb. It is unbelievable that medicinal plants give such results."

DIRECTION

Infusion: 1 heaped teaspoon per ¼ litre of boiling water, infused for a short time. Only 2 cups a day are taken, 1 cup in the morning on an empty stomach, 1 cup in the evening, half an hour before a meal.

WOOD SORREL (Oxalis acetosella)

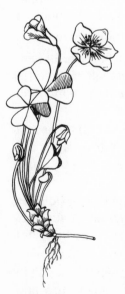

Common names are Wood Sour, Stickwort, Fairy Bells, Stubwort and Sour Trefoil.

It grows abundantly in woods where, with its light green leaves and dainty white flowers, it covers the ground like a blanket. This is very pleasing to the eye and when looking for mushrooms I sometimes nibble on a leaf. I gather the flowers in smaller amounts for a tea mixture (see page 60).

Wood Sorrel is not used dried but in a fresh state. It relieves **heartburn, stomach upsets and slight liver complaints**. For these, the tea is drunk cooled, 2 cups a day. For **jaundice, nephritis, eczema and worms** the same amount is drunk warm.

In popular medicine the freshly pressed juice is recommended for **stomach cancer in the early stage, cancer-like internal and external ulcers and growths**. Three to five drops diluted with water or tea are taken every hour. The freshly pressed juice is dabbed directly on external growths.

For the so called **shaking palsy (Parkinson's disease)** the juice, three to five drops in Yarrow tea, is sipped and, externally, rubbed into the spine. Dilutions and doses have to be adhered to conscientiously for stomach cancer, ulcers and growths, as well as for shaking palsy (Parkinson's disease).

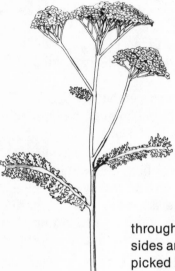

YARROW (Achillea millefolium)

Common names: Milfoil, Nosebleed, Soldier's Herb, Woundwort, Blood-wort and Knight's Milfoil.

Yarrow is a medicinal herb that would be difficult to be without; it is of great value for many illnesses but first and foremost, it is a herb for women. I cannot recommend Yarrow enough for women. Abbé Kneipp says in his writings: **"Women could be spared many troubles, if they just took Yarrow tea from time to time!"** Be it a young girl with **irregular menstruation** or an older woman during **menopause** or already past it, for everyone young and old, it is of importance to drink a cup of Yarrow tea from time to time. It is beneficial for the reproductive organs of women and they cannot do a better thing for their health than, while walking through the fields, pick some Yarrow. It grows in meadows and pastures, by road-sides and paths. The flowers are white or pink, have an aromatic smell and should be picked in bright sunshine, since the volatile oils and, therefore, their curative quality are greater.

It was said of a young woman that she had **cancer in the abdomen**. She received cobalt treatment. The relatives were told that there was no cure. I thought of the Abbé Kneipp and his advice for **abdominal disorders** and asked the woman to drink as much Yarrow tea as she could. I was surprised when after three weeks, I received a note saying she felt great and her weight was returning slowly but surely to normal.

For **inflammation of the ovaries** the first sitz bath will often relieve the pain and the inflammation will slowly subside. These sitz baths are also successful against **bedwetting** of children and older people, as well as **"whites"**. In these cases 2 cups of Yarrow tea should be drunk daily as well.

For **prolapse of the uterus** sitz baths are taken for a long time, 4 cups of Lady's Mantle tea are sipped daily and the area of the abdomen from the vagina upward is rubbed with Shepherd's Purse tincture.

For **fibroids** Yarrow sitz baths are taken until a medical check-up shows no sign of them anymore.

A girl of nineteen had not yet menstruated. A gynaecologist prescribed the pill for her. Her breasts became quite large but there was **no menstrual flow**. She refused to continue with the pill. Her mother came to see me and I told her to give the girl a cup of Yarrow tea on an empty stomach every morning. After 4 weeks everything was in order and the girl has had no problems since.

A woman during **menopause** should take advantage of Yarrow tea and save herself a lot of **inner restlessness** and other problems. Yarrow sitz baths are also good for the health. For **neuritis** in arms and legs, foot and arm baths with an addition of Yarrow are soothing, but the Yarrow has to be picked in the midday sun. These baths often relieve the pain after the first use.

Dr. Lutze recommends Yarrow tea for **"congestion in the head**, accompanied by terrible pain, **giddiness, nausea, running and weeping eyes, sharp pain in the eyes and nose bleeding . . ."** **Migraine**, caused by weather changes, is often relieved after only one cup of Yarrow tea which has to be sipped fairly hot. If the tea is drunk regularly, **migraine** can disappear completely.

In old herbals Yarrow is called "cure of all ills" and can be used in cases that seem hopeless. Through its **blood cleansing** action many an illness is expelled from the body. It is worth a try. That Yarrow acts directly and best on the **bone marrow** and thus stimulates **blood renewal**, is not well known. Yarrow is therefore helpful for **disorders of the bone marrow, even caries**, where other medication is of no avail, if the tea is drunk, baths are taken and a friction with Yarrow tincture is used. Yarrow is an excellent remedy for stopping **bleeding in the lungs** and used together with Calamus roots heals **lung cancer**. The Calamus roots are chewed throughout the day and a cup of Yarrow tea is sipped every morning and evening. The tea is beneficial for **bleeding haemorrhoids, stomach bleeding, indigestion and heartburn**. For **colds, back or rheumatic pain** Yarrow tea is drunk as hot as possible and in large amounts. The tea activates **sluggish kidneys, rectifies lack of appetite**, dispels **flatulence and stomach cramps**, is beneficial for **liver disorders, inflammation of the gastro-intestinal tract** and regulates the **movement of the bowels**.

Since the Yarrow helps in **circulatory disorders and vascular spasm**, it is recommended for **angina pectoris**. – Sitz baths or washing with a decoction of Yarrow relieve troublesome **itching in the vagina**.

An ointment is prepared from Yarrow flowers and used for **haemorrhoids**.

DIRECTIONS

Infusion: ¼ litre of boiling water is poured over 1 heaped teaspoon of herbs, infused for a short time.

Tincture: Yarrow flowers, picked in the sun, are placed loosely into a bottle. 38% to 40% rye whisky or wodka is poured over them and the bottle is left in the sun or in a warm place for 14 days.

Yarrow ointment: 90 gm. unsalted butter or lard are heated, 15 gm. freshly picked, cut Yarrow flowers and 15 gm. finely cut Raspberry leaves are added, stirred till crackling occurs and removed from the heat. The next day it is slightly warmed, pressed through a piece of linen, poured into clear jars and stored in the refrigerator.

Sitz bath: 100 gm. Yarrow (the whole herb) are steeped in cold water overnight. The next day brought to the boil and added to the bath water (see General Information "sitz bath").

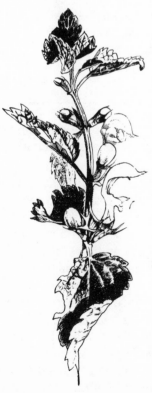

YELLOW DEAD NETTLE (Lamium galeobdolon)

Common names: Yellow Archangel, Dummy Nettle, Weazel Snout.

This plant grows in damp woods, in shady hedgerows, in waste places, quarries and wherever the Stinging Nettle grows. From the branched root stock the erect stems grow to a height of 50 cm. The pair of oval shaped, crenated leaves is placed exactly at right angles to the one above and below. The yellow flowers are arranged in whorls or rings in the axle of the leaves. The flowers and leaves are gathered.

Yellow Dead Nettle as well as **White Dead Nettle** (Lamium album) are valuable medicinal herbs. The latter flowers from May almost to December and is found as a common weed along paths, in waste places and on railway embankments. The leaves and especially the flowers are gathered. A tea is beneficial in **abdominal and menstrual complaints**, if 2 cups are sipped during the day. It cleanses the blood and is an effective remedy for **sleeplessness and for diverse female troubles**. People suffering from continual **abdominal complaints** and young girls should value this tea.

The leaves and flowers of the **Yellow Dead Nettle** are used for similar complaints, but especially for **scanty or burning urine, bladder trouble**, serious **kidney disorders and fluid retention in the heart**. The flowers are used for **digestive troubles, scrofula and skin rashes** and 1 cup of this tea is drunk during the morning. For **ulcers and varicose veins** compresses made from the infusion are beneficial. – Yellow Dead Nettle can be recommended for **bladder malfunction** with older people, as well as for **chill in the bladder and nephritis**. A sitz bath, with the decoction added, is very soothing.

For **cirrhosis of the kidneys and when renal dialysis** has to be performed, the Yellow Dead Nettle, Bedstraw and Golden Rod mixed in equal proportions, give good results.

DIRECTIONS (Yellow Dead Nettle)

Infusion: 1 heaped teaspoon per ¼ litre of boiling water, infused for a short time.

Compress: 3 heaped teaspoons per ½ litre of boiling water, infused for a short time. A cloth is soaked in the infusion and applied warmly.

Sitz bath: See General Information "sitz bath" (the whole plant is used).

Tea mixture: Yellow Dead Nettle, Bedstraw and Golden Rod in equal proportions are mixed. One heaped teaspoon per ¼ litre of boiling water.

***

SWEDISH HERBS

SMALL SWEDISH BITTERS

10 gm. Aloe*
5 gm. Myrrh
0,2 gm. Saffron
10 gm. Senna leaves ·
10 gm. Camphor**
10 gm. Rhubarb roots
10 gm. Zedvoary roots
10 gm. Manna
10 gm. Theriac venezian
5 gm. Carline Thistle roots
10 gm. Angelica roots

This mixture is put into a wide-necked 2 litre bottle and 1½ litre of 38% to 40% rye or fruit spirit are poured over it. The bottle is left standing in the sun or near the stove for 14 days and shaken daily. The liquid is then strained and poured into small bottles, well stoppered and stored in a cool place. This way it can be kept for many years. The longer it stands the more effective it becomes! Shake well before use! Alternatively some of the liquid can be strained into a small bottle and the rest left in the bottle until required.

* Instead of Aloe, Gentian root or Wormwood powder may be used.
** Only natural Camphor should be used.

This recipe was found among the writings of the well-known Swedish physician, rector of medicine, Dr. Samst. He died in his 104th year in a riding accident. His parents and grandparents all reached a patriarchal age.

It sounds almost like a fairy story, but it is true. As a refugee from the German speaking area of Czechoslovakia, I became ill with **typhoid fever** in a camp in Bavaria, caused by contaminated meat and, through it, came **jaundice and an obstruction in the intestines.** I spent more than 6 months in hospital and when my husband got my mother, my mother-in-law, our child and myself to Austria, I was a young but sick woman. At night I was hit by terrible pain that shot through my body like a sword. In these moments I could neither sit nor stand, walk nor lie down; at the same time I **vomited** and had **diarrhoea.** I was a helpless bundle of misery. These were **afterpains of the typhoid** fever which sometimes can go on for years, as the doctor said. One day a woman brought me a small bottle containing a dark brown, strong smelling liquid. She had heard of my illness and wanted to help. The Swedish Bitters had relieved her of a serious complaint. Accompanying it was a transcript of an **"old manuscript"** in which was explained, in 46 points, how these drops heal every illness. The recipe came from the writings of a well-known Swedish physician. As stated, all members of his family had reached an unusual old age. These drops, according to point 43 heal "plague boils and swellings even if already in the throat". I put the bottle in the medicine chest. I just did not believe that these modest drops could give me back my health, since the doctor could not even help me. Soon I changed my mind. As I sat in front of a large basket of over ripe pears which needed to be used up straight away I had another attack. As I had been told that these Swedish drops could be used externally as well, I did not hesitate for long and applied them as a compress on the abdomen, put a small plastic bag over the compress and then my girdle and continued my work. A wonderful warm feeling spread through my body and, suddenly, it felt as if with one movement of the hand, everything morbid in my body was pulled out. I assure you that with this single compress which I had on the whole day, all complaints of the preceding months disappeared, never to return.

When my son was 6 years old, he was attacked by an Alsatian and terribly mauled in the face. Later dark red scars covered his face from the nose upward. In the "old manuscript" point 33 states that this tincture takes away all **scars, wounds and cuts**, even if very old, if moistened up to 40 times. Therefore our son's scars were now moistened daily. Very soon they disappeared, even the ones deep in the nose.

With these experiences I came to our town in 1953. During a visit to a farmhouse I met the farmer's wife, a mother of 2 small children, milking the cows. Instead of a word of greeting she said: "If you stood me against the wall I would let you shoot me." For weeks she had suffered from terrible **headaches** and she was supposed to go for X-rays. The same evening I sent my son with a small bottle of Swedish Bitters to her, so that she might find relief, at least at night. How surprised I was when, at 7 o'clock in the morning, the farmer came to me saying: "What did you send my wife? Within a short time, after applying it to the head, the headaches had gone. And in the morning 2 dark brown clots of the thickness of a little finger came down her throat." This woman swears by the Swedish Bitters even today and was able to help her little daughter who suffered from **pneumonia** years ago. Never is she without this household remedy.

For months, a woman suffered from **frontal sinusitis**. She could not breathe through her nose and was plagued by terrible headaches. Despite antibiotics and radiation treatment her condition did not improve. Then she applied Swedish Bitters as a compress over the forehead, eyes and nose and already after the first use she felt relief. 3 nightly treatments later, large amounts of pus came through her nose and she was able to breathe normally again.

From sight I knew a young woman who after the birth of her sixth child became a shadow of herself. I spoke to her and learned that at this time she **was unable to eat anything** and was also unable to keep the children with her. I recommended Swedish Bitters to her. About 3 weeks later I saw her as a healthy young woman who was able to eat normally and had the children with her again. Her mother had been in hospital with a swollen foot and for a long time had only been able to walk with a stick. Despite 75 injections there was no improvement. Therefore this young woman sent the recipe of the Swedish Bitters to her mother, advising her to try them. Now her mother's foot is back to normal and the stick unnecessary.

One day, I received a letter from Germany in which an acquaintance asked me to look after her niece who was taking a cure in Gallspach. When the young woman came to see me for the first time, I got a shock. She was lifted out of the car, crutches were put under her arms and it took her, despite help, more than an hour to come up into my flat on the first floor. The joints of both feet were deformed, the fingers crippled and unable to hold anything. When walking, the **body was thrown** forward and the legs pulled after. I stood at the door, my hands pressed against my heart, unable to say anything except: "How does a young woman like you have such a terrible illness?" "Overnight after my fourth child", she replied. Quite suddenly, almost overnight, this young woman lay crippled in her bed. She was taken from doctor to doctor, nobody could help her. Twice a year she came to Gallspach to Dr. Zeileis who had to tell her he could not cure her, only ease the trouble. I recommended Swedish Bitters and told her to put her faith in it. This was in February, 1964. In September I received a telephone call from the young woman, asking if I could meet her at the bus stop. I was baffled, then surprised, when a smiling young woman, still leaning on a stick, descended the bus. The **stiffness and crippling of the hands** was gone, as well as some of the **deformation of the legs**. Only on the left foot, the knee and the ankle were still swollen. But on the third of August, 1965, a year later, this too had disappeared completely and she came without a stick, a healthy woman to take the cure for the last time. She had put 1 tablespoon of Swedish Bitters 3 times daily into a small amount of lukewarm water and sipped it before and after each meal.

I would like to give a few more examples of the wonderful effect of Swedish Bitters. From my sister who lives in Germany I learned that a mutual acquaintance from Leipzig had been confined to a wheelchair for 15 years. She had spent the war years in Praque and in 1945 — as was the fate of many — had to stay for weeks in a cellar without straw or any other bedding. Later she came to Leipzig with her husband. Soon she suffered from terrible **deformations of the joints** and then came the life in a wheelchair. I only learned of her difficult fate when her husband suddenly died and the poor **crippled woman** had to leave the flat and move into a furnished room. The sending of herbs or medications from Austria to East Germany is not allowed, therefore I had to send her the herb mixture from a border town in Bavaria every second month. Soon I received encouraging letters. She took 1 tablespoon of Swedish Bitters in a small amount of water and drank half of it before and half of it after a meal. She did this 3 times a day. Slowly the deformations receded and she was able to move her joints slightly. We prayed, she in Leipzig, we in Austria. After 9 months, this woman who had been tied to a wheelchair for 15 years, could leave her flat for the first time. Slowly she improved and was soon able to do her daily work which helpful people had so far done for her.

In the summer we often went swimming in a lake. One day, the large piece of wood that we used to sit on was leaning against a fence. I had my bag next to it and was bending over to gather up some things, when all of a sudden I felt this terrific blow on my leg. The large piece of timber had fallen over and struck me right on the leg. In no time, from the knee downward, it was dark blue to purple and two large swellings, about the size of a first, appeared. I was carried to the car and then up to my room. My husband wanted to send for the doctor, but I asked him to apply Swedish Bitters as a compress on my leg. Half an hour later I was able to walk down the stairs to the dining room without help. The next day my leg was smooth, there were no more swellings and the **discolouration** had cleared up as well.

Another accident happened near this lake. A 4 year old girl was stung by a **hornet** and her arm swelled up. I fetched Swedish Bitters and before the parents had clothed the girl, I was ready with the compress and applied it while the girl was carried to the car. On arrival at the car, about 3 minutes later, the **swelling** had subsided and the doctor was no longer necessary.

While gathering raspberries, I was stung by a **poisonous insect** in the thumb. Overnight the thumb swelled up and while shopping a woman said to me: "You had better go directly to hospital, such an infection could cause your death." Overnight I applied Swedish Bitters as a compress and the next day my thumb was back to its normal size.

One time I had an accident in the laundry. It was at the time when washing machines washed but did not rinse. The heavily entangled pieces had to be lifted out of the very hot water with wooden tongs. I tend to do everything quickly and with great energy. The tongs slipped and hit me in the eye. Stunned with pain and half blind I walked upstairs. As soon as I had applied Swedish Bitters, the terrible pain eased. A little while later, I looked into the mirror and saw that I had given myself a **black eye**. I was back in the laundry a quarter of an hour later with a piece of cotton wool moistened with Swedish Bitters covering the eye, a small piece of plastic over it and the whole lot tied up with a folded scarf. For a few days I kept applying these compresses overnight, thence there was no chance of anything developing behind the eye.

As I do every year, I was taking a cure in a Kneipp Spa in Mühllacken, when the head nurse came into my room with a woman doubled up with pain. She suffered from **gallbladder attacks** and the doctor had advised her to have an operation. I applied Swedish Bitters as a compress on the area of the gall bladder (first Calendula ointment or lard has to be applied otherwise the alcohol would dry out the skin, then a piece of cotton wool is moistened with Swedish Bitters, applied to the **painful area**, a piece of dry cotton wool and a piece of plastic are put over it to keep it warm. Everything is now bandaged with a piece of cloth). I was just about to pull up her girdle when she sat up with a cry: "The pain is gone!" She continued to apply the compresses and she took the Swedish Bitters as drops, internally, 3 times a day, one teaspoonful in a little water or tea and the attacks never reoccurred.

For years I looked after a woman who was all alone. Communication with her was somewhat difficult, since she was **hard of hearing**. In the "old manuscript" it says: **"They bring back lost hearing."** Therefore she had to moisten the acoustic duct frequently with Swedish Bitters. The index finger, moistened with Swedish Bitters, is put into the ear. Do not forget to put a drop of oil into the ear from time to time, to avoid itching. At the same time this woman moistened her temples, her forehead and the area around the eyes. Now we can communicate normally and her face has a much fresher look. One day, as she was getting out of the bus, a car knocked her down and she fell on her face. Again Swedish Bitters helped her blue-red face to get back its normal colour. On February 1st, she celebrated her 89th birthday. How often have people who come to my talks told me that they are able to hear again and have packed away their hearing aid thanks to Swedish Bitters. These drops relieve pain internally or externally, anywhere in the body, because the blood supply to the affected area is increased. Therefore it is appropriate to apply Swedish Bitters as a compress to the back of the head of people who suffer from **epileptic fits**. The cause of these attacks lies often back in the past; maybe a fall on the head or a shock in childhood.

During a talk I gave, a man came up to me and told me that he received a double fracture of the base of the scull in a very bad car accident. After this had healed he started to get a few **epileptic fits** a day. I recommended Swedish Bitters applied as a compress to the back of the head, and 4 cups of Stinging Nettle tea, to which 2 tablespoons of Swedish Bitters were added, daily. Stinging Nettle tea is necessary for severe epileptic fits. Several months later he passed by my house to tell me that the fits had stopped.

Meningitis, head injuries caused by a **fall or a blow, stuttering and speech disorders** are treated effectively with Swedish Bitters applied as a compress to the back of the head. These compresses are also beneficial for **bursitis**. I have to emphasize again that for all severe illnesses a doctor has to be consulted first!

From the many letters I have received I have learnt that Swedish Bitters applied as a compress to the eyes has been effective in cases of a **detached retina and porous retina**. All these people were going blind. These compresses are applied to the closed eye and left on for an hour. **Healthy** eyes, especially if **strained**, can profit too, if Swedish Bitters is brushed with the index finger along the lid to the corner of the eye. This way good **eye sight** can be enjoyed well into old age.

Since Swedish Bitters is such a wonderful remedy, no medicine chest in the house should be without it. Poured into small bottles it can be taken along on trips. Often away from home, the food is disappointing and the need arises to **stimulate digestion** and to shake off **weariness and tiredness**. In these cases Swedish Bitters is a true "elixir". A sip, watered down, is taken internally and, externally, some drops are brushed on temples, forehead, eyes and the area behind the ears. In no time the beneficial effect is felt.

For a **cold**, with all its accompanying symptoms such as weariness, tiredness, pressure in the head and heaviness in the stomach, a cotton ball is moistened with Swedish Bitters and held under the nose, while breathing in deeply. Immediately the head feels lighter. If the **cold** has already affected the **bronchial** tubes, the moistened cotton ball is held in front of the open mouth and breathing in is done with the mouth. Here, too, relief will be felt. During times of influenza, 1 teaspoon, sometimes 1 tablespoon, diluted with a little water, is taken daily. In this way one is protected from the influenza. Wherever there is **pain**, Swedish Bitters is always beneficial, taken internally as drops, applied as a compress or used as a rub or massage.

Several years ago I suffered from **renal colic**. The doctor came in the middle of his surgery hours. In the meantime I had applied Swedish Bitters as a compress on the kidney region and when the doctor arrived the pain had subsided. I was quite shame-faced because I had wasted his valuable time. He wanted to know why the pain had subsided so quickly. When he heard that I had applied a compress he said: "Excellent, I do not have to give you an injection!" Swedish Bitters had his approval. Whenever I came to his surgery he would say: **"I will not prescribe you anything, you have Swedish Bitters."** It was he who had brought me closer to herbs.

An elderly lady came to see me. For years she could only walk with a stick, since **arthritis** had crippled her; nothing helped and she could not take it any longer. 1 teaspoon of Swedish Bitters in Stinging Nettle tea and Horsetail tea, taken 3 times a day, made a difference and 3 weeks later I heard she was able to walk without a stick.

A member of our small church choir **injured her knee** while ice skating. Since it was a small choir she was missed badly. After church I met her in town. It was impossible for her to mount the steep staircase up to the choir. A few moments later I was at her place with the things required for a compress. As a doctor's wife she looked sceptically at my doings. This changed when she was able to bend her knee a few minutes later and the next day she was able to mount the staircase. But unfortunately another member was missing, due to a **sprained ankle** acquired while enjoying our so healthy wintersport. We knew that she was already at the casualty ward. Now the lady who only the day before had had a **stiff knee** asked me to go and put the compress on the sprained ankle. I was reluctant to do it, because the woman had been treated at the hospital, but thinking I might find myself singing alone I changed my mind. I found her lying on the couch with a very swollen, painful **ankle**. In the hospital she was told just to keep her foot raised. Swedish Bitters applied as a compress brought her immediately some relief. The next day she came to the choir, although the roads were icy. She was without pain and her ankle was normal.

One day in a restaurant I saw a man who was obviously in pain. I got out my Swedish Bitters and gave him a tablespoonful in a little luke-warm water. Colour came back to his face and he could not believe it when the pain subsided. 6 months later I came back to the same place, I had already forgotten the incident, when a gentleman came up and thanked me profusely. He looked years younger. With the help of Swedish Bitters he had lost all complaints which **acute gastritis and disorder of the pancreas** had caused him. Since Swedish Bitters clears up disorders of the pancreas, they are most beneficial for **diabetes. Warts, liver spots, corns, moles, haemorrhoids even birthmarks and seborrhoea** will disappear, if they are moistened repeatedly with Swedish Bitters. A piece of cotton wool moistened with Swedish Bitters, put in the ear, will clear up **buzzing and ringing**. If the base of the scalp is moistened, it will **strengthen the memory**. Swedish Bitters cleanses the **blood, improves circulation, dispels flatulence, headaches, indigestion, stomach, gallbladder, liver and kidney disorders** (even if alcohol is not allowed). For **phlebitis and thrombosis**, Calendula ointment is smeared thickly on the affected areas and then Swedish Bitters, as a compress, is applied. When healed, Stinging Nettle foot baths are taken to improve the circulation. These drops stimulate a **sluggish intestine** and dispel **dizziness and lameness**. For all illnesses they are most beneficial, even for **cancer**. For acute attacks of pain, 1 tablespoonful is taken in a little water or tea. If 1 teaspoonful in a little water is taken 3 times daily, morning, noon and evening, good health is kept till old age. Swedish Bitters awakens vitality and strengthens the life force so needed in our time. Preserve through them your health, strength and joy for your family, work and fellowman.

During a visit at a farm I heard that the 12 year old son was to have an operation. **Pus** had formed behind the ear drum, due to an inflammation. I was against an operation, since sometimes, in similar cases, deafness occurs. A small piece of cotton wool moistened with Swedish Bitters was put in the boy's ear. A lot of pus was discharged daily, the pain subsided and an operation was not necessary.

For **intestinal cancer** – it was a young mother of five and the doctor had given her only a few more days – I recommended compresses applied to the area of the intestines, at the same time Calamus roots which are steeped in cold water overnight (1 level teaspoon per cup of water); 1 sip before and after each meal, and a tea made from equal proportions of Stinging Nettle, Calendula and Yarrow. At least 2 litres of this tea have to be sipped throughout the day. Today this woman is so much better that there is hope of a complete recovery.

A woman from Heilbronn, West Germany wrote: "About 10 months ago, my 41 year old nephew who lives in Sacramento, California, wrote in his letter that he suffers from **bleeding of the colon** daily and the medical diagnosis is without doubt **cancer of the colon**. A side opening would be necessary. I sent him your book 'Health through God's Pharmacy', Swedish Bitters, Calamus roots, Calendula, Yarrow and Stinging Nettle. He followed the instructions in your book. Today my nephew is able to work again. After taking the mentioned herbs for 4 days the bleeding stopped. Tiredness and loss of weight were arrested slowly."

A 52 year old man treated for 10 years for **cardiac asthma**, had to take 8 tablets daily. For years he could only sleep sitting up and, for every step he took, he had to throw up his arms to get some air. I was of the opinion that this was caused not by the heart but the liver. I applied Swedish Bitters as a compress to the area of the liver. He had to drink 1 cup of Common Club Moss tea to which a teaspoon of Swedish Bitters had been added in the morning and the same in the evening, daily. How right I was showed the first night, when he was able to sleep lying down. Swedish Bitters and Common Club Moss tea brought about a swift and good improvement, so that, 3 days later, he who had not stepped out of his house for years was able to walk around his little garden twice during the day. Slowly he is recovering.

A **wound** which would not heal after an operation closed overnight, after the patient had taken a large sip of the bottle of Swedish Bitters. This single sip caused the wound to close which had been open for three years and had to be dressed several times a day.

A lady from Burgenland, Austria, told me that her 23 year old niece had an **auditory defect** since birth. She was told that an operation in her case would be without success. This lady then asked her niece to try Swedish Bitters. They were very surprised when, 14 days later, the niece was able to hear normally.

My dear readers, I do not want to withhold a letter from Graz, Styria: "By chance or maybe Providence, I had a talk with a 74 year old man in the bus. This man got back his hearing which he had lost during the war, when receiving **head and brain injuries**. Only 3 times had he put a piece of cotton wool moistened with Swedish Bitters in his ears." (Letters provide the proof of such accounts.)

A gentleman from Bavaria reports: "Through an accident I **injured my right arm**. Swedish Bitters soon alleviated the terrible pain. After almost 10 years of **deafness** in one ear, I was able to hear the ticking of the alarm clock again. Only twice did I put Swedish Bitters into my ear." – How many **deaf** people could be helped this way! Even if only a single one could get back his hearing.

After a talk I gave, I learned from a listener that, for 2 years, she had suffered from a **weak anus muscle**. The doctor said it was irreparable. Swedish Bitters, together with Shepherd's Purse, finely cut, macerated in rye whisky or wodka and kept in a warm place for 10 days, heals muscular atrophy and serious muscular disorders; four cups of Lady's Mantle tea and six sips of Calamus root tea a day remedied it.

In a telephone call from Vienna I heard a female voice say: **"Thank you so much for Swedish Bitters."** When 12 years old, during a school hike in the mountains, this woman was inadvertently hit in the face by the girl in front of her with her climbing boot. Hence, for 40 years, of and on, she suffered from a **festering jaw** and had undergone 16 operations and several punctures. She had to break off her studies, was unable to take the profession she wanted and plagued by continuous pain, she looked after a household. When 52 years old she read about Swedish Bitters, applied it as a compress on the jaw area and finally was freed from all pain.

Again and again I receive inquiries, if Swedish Bitters can be used, when **alcohol is prohibited**. According to credible laboratory tests, the **herbs drown the alcohol and are considered as medicine**. Therefore they can be taken without detriment. In such a case, first of all commence with 1 teaspoon a day and a compress should be applied to the area of the kidney and liver (see "directions" at the end of this chapter).

"OLD MANUSCRIPT" (Transcript of the Swedish Bitters' curative power)

1. If they are frequently breathed in or sniffed, the base of the scull is moistened or a moistened cloth applied to the head, they dispel **pain and dizziness** and strengthen the brain and **memory**.
2. They help dim eyes and take away redness and all pain, even if the **eyes are inflamed**. They rid them of **spots and cataracts**, if the corners are moistened in time or a moistened piece of cloth is applied to the closed lids.
3. **Pustulas and eczema** of all kinds, as **scabs** in the nose or elsewhere on the body, are healed, if they are often and well moistened.
4. For **toothache** a tablespoon of these drops is taken with a little water and kept in the mouth for a little while or the aching tooth is moistened. The pain soon eases and the putrefaction disappears.
5. **Blisters on the tongue** or other infirmities of the tongue are frequently moistened with the drops and healing soon occurs.
6. If the **throat is hot or inflamed**, so that food is only **swallowed with difficulty**, these drops are swallowed slowly, morning, noon and evening and they take away the heat and heal the throat.
7. For **stomach cramps**, 1 tablespoonful is taken.
8. For **colic**, 3 tablespoonsfull are taken slowly, one after the other, and relief will soon be felt.
9. They rid the body of **wind (gas)** and cool the liver, eliminate all troubles of the intestines and stomach and help **constipation**.
10. An excellent remedy for **stomach disorders**, if the **digestion** is faulty or food cannot be kept down.
11. They are beneficial for **pain in the gall bladder**. 1 tablespoonful daily in the morning and evening and, at night, compresses and soon all pain will disappear.
12. For **dropsy** 1 tablespoonful in white wine is taken in the morning and evening for 6 weeks.
13. For **pain and buzzing in the ear** a piece of cotton wool is moistened and put into the ear. It is very beneficial and brings back **lost hearing**.
14. For **morning sickness**, 1 tablespoon of the drops in red wine is given in the morning for 3 days, half an hour later a walk is taken, then breakfast, but no milk. These drops should not be taken after drinking milk.
15. In the last 14 days of **pregnancy** if 1 tablespoon of the drops is taken mornings and evenings, it **promotes the birth**. For easy **expelling of the afterbirth**, a coffeespoonful is given every 2 hours, until the afterbirth is expelled without pain.
16. If, after a birth when the **milk dries up**, inflammation develops, it quickly subsides if a moistened piece of cloth is applied.
17. They expel **worms**, even **tapeworms**, in children and adults, the amount taken by children being according to age. A piece of cloth moistened with drops is applied to the navel and kept moist.

18. They rid children of **pustulas**. The children are given these drops according to age, diluted with water. If the pustulas start to dry up they are moistened frequently with these drops and no scars will develop.

19. For **jaundice** very soon all complaints disappear, if 1 tablespoon of these drops is taken 3 times daily and compresses are applied to the **swollen liver**.

20. They open all **haemorrhoids**, heal the **kidneys**, rid the body of all unnecessary liquids without further treatment, taking away **melancholy and depression** and improve appetite and digestion.

21. **Haemorrhoids** are reduced, if, in the beginning, they are moistened frequently and if the drops are taken internally, especially before going to bed, they soften the haemorrhoids. Externally a cotton ball moistened with the drops is applied. It makes the remaining blood flow and relieves the burning.

22. If someone has **fainted**, open his mouth if required, give him 1 tablespoon of the drops and he will come to.

23. This remedy rids you of the pain of **spasm** (cramps) so that it will cease in time.

24. For **consumption** take them daily in the morning on an empty stomach and continue the treatment for 6 weeks.

25. If the **menstrual flow ceases** for a woman or it is too heavy, she takes these drops 3 days and repeats it 20 times. They will, what is too much, quieten and, what is too little, even out.

26. This remedy also helps to cure **"whites" (white vaginal discharge)**.

27. If someone is afflicted with **epilepsy**, he has to be given these drops on the spot and he should then take this remedy exclusively, since it strengthens the affected nerves as well as the body and rids it of all sickness.

28. They heal **lameness** and rid you of **dizziness and indisposition**.

29. They heal also hot **pustulas and erysipelas**.

30. If someone has **fever**, be it hot or could, and is very weak, he is given 1 tablespoonful of the drops and the patient, if he is not overloaded with other medications, will in a short time come to, the pulse will start to beat again and the fever, no matter how high it was, will pass and the patient will soon be better.

31. The drops also heal **cancer, old pock marks, warts and chapped hands**. If the wound is **old or festering or proud flesh** has developed, everything is washed well with white wine and a piece of cloth moistened with the drops is laid upon it.

32. They heal, without danger, all **wounds**, be they from a stab or a hit, if they are moistened frequently. A piece of cloth is taken, moistened with the drops and the wounds covered therewith. They take away the pain in a short time, permit no **blemish or putrefication** and heal also old wounds which were caused by a **shot**. If there are holes, the drops are sprinkled into the wound which need not necessarily be cleaned beforehand. Through repeated applying of the moistened cloth healing occurs in a short time.

33. They take away **scars**, even if very old, **wounds and cuts** if moistened up to 40 times with them. All the wounds heal and leave no scars.

34. They heal all **fistulas**, even if they seem incurable, be they as old as may be.

35. They heal all **burns and scalds**, be they caused by fire, hot water or fat, if the injuries are moistened frequently. No blisters form, the heat is taken out and even festering blisters are healed.

36. They serve against **swellings and bruises**, be they caused by a blow or a fall.

37. If someone cannot eat with **appetite**, they bring back the lost taste.

38. In **anaemia** they bring back the lost colour, if taken for a period in the morning. They cleanse the blood and form new blood and promote circulation.

39. **Rheumatic pains** in the limbs are eased if the drops are taken morning and evening and a moistened cloth is applied to the aching parts.

40. They heal **frost bitten hands and feet**, even if there are open parts, if a moistened cloth is applied as often as possible, but especially at night.

41. For **corns**, a cotton ball, moistened with the drops, is applied and kept moist. After 3 days the corns fall out or can be removed painlessly.

42. They heal too **bites** of mad dogs and other animals, if taken internally, since they heal and destroy all poison. A moistened cloth is laid upon the wounds.

43. For **plague** and other **infectious diseases** it is well to take them repeatedly since they heal **plague boils and swellings** even if already in the throat.

44. He who cannot sleep at night takes these drops before going to bed. For nervous **sleeplessness** a piece of cloth moistened with diluted drops is laid upon the heart.

45. A **drunk** can be sober on the spot with 2 tablespoonfuls.

46. He who takes these drops mornings and evenings daily needs no further medication, since they strengthen the body, tone up the nerves and the blood, take away the **trembling of hands and feet**. In short, they take away all illness. The body stays supple, the face young and beautiful.

Important: All stated amounts of Swedish Bitters should be taken diluted with herb tea or water.

The wonderful healing power of this herb mixture is shown in the above text of the "old manuscript". It can be said, and rightly so, that there is hardly any illness where Swedish Bitters is not of benefit, or at least is effective as a basis for every treatment.

DIRECTIONS

Internally: Prophylactics are taken according to the "old manuscript" in the morning and evening, 1 teaspoonful diluted with water. For indisposition of any kind, 3 tablespoons diluted with water can be taken. For serious diseases, 2 to 3 tablespoons are taken as follows: 1 tablespoon diluted with half a cup of herb tea, half of it is sipped half an hour before and the other half an hour after each meal.

Compress: According to area, a piece of cotton wool or gauze is moistened with Swedish Bitters and applied to the affected area which has been well covered with lard or Calendula ointment. A slightly larger piece of plastic is put over it to prevent the clothes from getting stained. Then a cloth is wound around or a bandage is used.

The compress can be left on, depending on illness, for 2 to 4 hours. If tolerated, the compress can stay on overnight. After removal the skin is powdered. Should people with sensitive skin still develop a rash, the compresses have to be used for a shorter period only or omitted for a time. People who are allergic to plastic should leave it off. Never forget to grease the skin beforehand. If an itching rash has already developed it can be treated with Calendula ointment.

GREAT SWEDISH BITTERS

Despite repeated suggestions I could not bring myself to write the recipe of the Great Swedish Bitters in this book, since all my successes have been achieved with the Small Swedish Bitters. This does not mean that the Great Swedish Bitters would be used less successfully.

HEART WINE

No Christian household should be without Dr. Hertzka's booklet "God heals" (St. Hildegard von Bingen's Medicine as a new natural course of treatment), published by Christiana-Verlag, Stein/Rhein (Switzerland). In it is cited among other things a great recipe which brings exceptionally good results for people suffering from a heart condition.

The Abbess Hildegard von Bingen, who lived 800 years ago (1098 – 1179), died in her 81st year. As a so-called mystic, she had, while totally awake, visions before her eyes. As she explicitly testified and declared before her death, everything she had ever written originated from these heavenly pictures and words. All mentioned illnesses and described medications were revealed to her by God.

Pope Eugen III had her gift of vision verified and her charisma acknowledged by the church. Now, 800 years later, her medical knowledge has been recognized also by modern medicine.

Dr. Hertzka, General Practitioner in Constance, Lake Constance, has given us the recipe for the heart wine in one of his books.

This heart wine shows very great success in all **disorders of the heart and cardiac weaknesses** and, as Dr. Hertzka says, is of much impotance in his daily practice. I, myself, have passed on this recipe several times and the success was surprisingly good. For **angina pectoris** this wine gives noticeable relief.

RECIPE FOR HEART WINE

10 freshly picked **Parsley stems** with leaves are put into 1 litre of pure wine, 2 tablespoons of **wine vinegar** are added. This is simmered for 10 minutes on low heat (careful, it foams). Then 300 gm. of pure **honey** are added and everything is slightly boiled for 4 minutes, strained and, still hot, bottled. The bottles have to be rinsed beforehand with strong alcohol. Well stoppered. The sediment that forms does not harm and can be drunk.

Dr. Hertzka says: "Which wine you take, be it red or white is of no importance, only it has to be pure... Only the order has to be adhered to. The honey is added after the first boiling and has to be boiled, too. Don't be afraid of boiling... So boil yourself the Parsley-honey wine, so beneficial to the heart."

Dr. Hertzka continues: "When your heart troubles you, take 1, 2 or even 3 or more tablespoonsful of this wine a day, and all **pains in the heart**, caused by a change of the weather or excitement, will disappear as if blown away. You need not be anxious or afraid, because you cannot do any harm. Not only for slight pain in the heart, but also for **cardiac weakness** and real **heart trouble**, this Parsley-honey wine will do you a great service, maybe even bring about a recovery."

On January 21st, 1980, I received a letter from Salzburg which I would like to quote: "I want to tell you that I have prepared the wine and that I have obtained amazing results. 10 years ago I was operated on and told that I have a **weak heart** and therefore will always have pain, nothing could be done about it and I would have to accept it. But thanks to the wine all my complaints have vanished. After taking this Parsley-honey wine for 2 months I do not feel weak anymore."

An excellent TEA MIXTURE for the family table

In early spring the gathering is started with the first flowers of Coltsfoot and continued on throughout the seasons with what nature provides continuously:

Coltsfoot flowers, later the leaves
Cowslip (flower heads)
Violets (flowers and leaves)
Lungwort (flowerheads)
Wood Sorrel (flowers)
Ground Ivy, a small amount only — as a flavouring
Stinging Nettle, the first young shoots in spring
Lady's Mantle (leaves and flowers)
Speedwell (flowers, stems and leaves)
Strawberry leaves, **Blackberry** and **Raspberry** shoots
Elder shoots, later flowers
Daisy
Linden flowers (picked in sunshine)
Camomile (picked in the sun)

Goat's Beard flowers (Tragopogon pratensis)
Calendula or Marigold (flowers)
Woodruff (stems, leaves and flowers)
Thyme (flowers, leaves and stems)
Balm Mint (stems, leaves and flowers or without flowers)
Peppermint (stems, leaves and flowers or without flowers)
Yarrow (only a small amount – picked in the sun)
Mullein (flowers – picked in the sun)
St. John's Wort (flowers – picked in the sun)
Marjoram (flowers and leaves)
Small Flowered Willow-herb (leaves, stems and flowers)
Fir (very young shoots)
Galium (flowers, leaves and stems)
Rose petals in all colours (only organically grown)

The herbs are dried well and in late autumn mixed to make a delicious tea. It will enrich your evening meal in winter and remind you of the beautiful summer hours you have spent. 1 heaped teaspoon per cup of boiling water is used and infused for a short time.

For personal notes:

ADVICE FOR VARIOUS DISORDERS

ACNE

These pimply eruptions plague many young people during puberty and are partly caused by kidney trouble. For this reason strongly spiced, salted dishes and acid salads and drinks should be avoided. Salads should be prepared with sour cream. For acne 1 litre of **Stinging Nettle** tea should be sipped throughout the day.

External application: A **Horseradish vinegar** is applied to the wet face and left on for ten minutes mornings and evenings. The shredded Horseradish is put into a bottle and wine or fruit vinegar is poured over it until the Horseradish is covered. This is left standing in a temperate room. Since it is used directly from the bottle without being strained, a sterilized plastic bottle with a perforated lid should be used. The Horseradish takes away the sharpness of the vinegar, the vinegar the hotness of the Horse-radish, the result is a mild vinegar essence easily tolerated by the facial skin.

AMPUTATION ("ghost pain")

Long after, sometimes years after, an amputation, "ghost pain" still occurs. Experiences show that **Comfrey poultices** (see chapter on Comfrey "directions" page 19) bring some easing and gradually the pain disappears.

Onion essence which can be bought at homoeopathic chemists is also effective. It can be easily pre-pared. A bottle is filled up to the neck with Onions sliced into rings; 38% to 40% rye whisky or wodka is poured over them and the bottle is left to stand in the sun or in a warm place for 10 days, then the liquid is strained and bottled. This essence is rubbed on the amputation stump.

Of great benefit is a tea made of the **roots of the Iris** which are dug up in October, are thoroughly cleaned and hung up to dry. The dried roots are ground (a coffee grinder will do). One ½ teaspoonful of this powder is soaked in a cup of water overnight; 1 to 2 cups are sipped during the day.

The amputation stump should be bathed in an infusion of **Thyme** 3 times a week (the water can be warmed and re-used twice); 1 handful of Thyme per bath is used. — **Thyme and Common Club Moss pillows**, applied overnight, are recommended. 100 gm. to 150 gm. of the mentioned herbs are filled into a linen bag.

APPENDIX, irritation of

"If a cup of freshly picked **Blackberry leaves** tea was drunk once in a while, there never would be an irritation of the appendix." This saying of my childhood's family doctor I remembered, when, one mor-ning, my 7 year old son awoke, looking very pale and feeling pain in the region of the appendix. I rang for the doctor and prepared a cup of Blackberry leaves tea immediately and gave it to my son to drink. His colour soon returned and when the doctor arrived he could not find any sign of an irritation of the appendix.

APPETITE, lack of (in children)

A young mother complained that her 2 year old son suffered from a chronic lack of appetite, was tired and listless, had dark rings under the eyes and hardly ever wanted to go for a walk. This changed rapidly when, following my advice, she gave the child a **Thyme bath** which was prepared from 50 gm of herbs (see chapter on Thyme "directions"; the heart region has to be outside the water). In addition the child had to sip 1 cup of **Stinging Nettle tea** daily. The happy mother told me that she hardly recognized her child. He showed good appetite, enjoyed being outdoors and going for walks. It was quite funny, how the little boy kept reminding her of the Stinging Nettle tea "one sip at a time" as he said.

ARTHROSIS AND ARTHRITIS

The following suggestions hold good also for inflamed and deformed joints and wear and tear symptoms. They can be remedied; the pain will subside slowly, even deformations recede gradually in the course of 1 to 2 years. People who have to use crutches or canes are able to put them away in a relatively short time. 1 cup of **Horsetail** tea left to infuse for ½ minute is drunk half an hour before breakfast and 1 cup before the evening meal, as well as 4 cups of **Stinging Nettle** tea. Of these 4 cups, ½ cup is taken off to which is added 1 tablespoon of **Swedish Bitters**. This is done 3 times a day and sipped before and after each meal.

Wherever pain occurs, in the knee or in other joints, Swedish Bitters are applied as a compress for four hours. Do not forget to grease the skin beforehand with Calendula ointment and to powder it afterwards, so that no itching occurs. **Crinkly cabbage or Cabbage leaves**, heated with an iron, applied and kept warm with a piece of cloth, bring relief.

A massage with **Comfrey tincture** is beneficial. For inflamed joints **Horsetail poultices** (p. 29) are used.

Besides Cabbage leaves, the leaves of **Cow-parsnip** or Hogweed (Heracleum sphondylium) are recommended. This plant is found in meadows, on banks and has large umbels, greenish to light pink.

Our granny, 93 years old, suddenly developed a painful **protrusion on the** right side of her left **knee**. Normally very agile, she had to use a cane and, even so, could hardly walk with it. I applied Swedish Bitters as a compress (4 hours) during the day and Cabbage leaves, heated with an iron, at night, for 14 days. The pain subsided somewhat, but she still had trouble walking. Then I gathered Cow-parsnip leaves, washed them and crushed them on a wooden board and applied them directly on the knee overnight. The next day, she was able to walk, only the protrusion was still noticeable. I repeated the application and next day it was gone, too. Now 94 years old, our granny still walks without a cane.

Recommended are **Horsetail sitz baths** once a month; 100 gm. herbs are steeped in cold water overnight and warmed in the morning. The bath should last for 20 minutes. The bath water can be poured back over the herbs, warmed and re-used twice.

A nun wrote: "In April I asked for your advice. I could hardly sleep at night because of pain. As recommended, I have drunk 3 cups of tea made from freshly picked Stinging Nettles to which I added 1 tablespoon of Swedish Bitters. I have to tell you with great pleasure that now, 6 months later, I have no pain in my hip and require no operation. Since I work in a home for old people, I have been able to help many an old person by using herbs."

ATROPHY OF THE BONES

The ground seeds of **Fenugreek** are used successfully for this disease, as well as for **osteo-myelitis and bone growth**. One half cup of **Yarrow tea** is drunk 4 times a day and to 2 of these half cups ½ a teaspoon of ground Fenugreek seeds is added. Yarrow baths, 200 gm. herbs per bath (the water can be re-used twice), should be taken for 20 minutes once a month. The heart region should be outside the water. Yarrow tincture is rubbed into the body (see "directions" under Yarrow).

BAD BREATH – FURRED TONGUE

Bad breath is not only unpleasant for the one concerned, but also for his fellow man. First of all a medical check-up should establish the cause of it. It could be **bad teeth, ulcers in the mouth, tonsillitis, secretion** of the mucous membrane **of the nose**, not enough **stomach acid or constipation**. For the latter it means, first of all, to bring about a regulated digestion.

For ulcers in the mouth gargling with warm **Bedstraw tea** is recommended, and for tonsillitis, with **Sage tea**. For secretion of the mucous membrane of the nose, Sage tea is sniffed up the nose. Often a few drops of **Juniper oil** in a glass of lukewarm water, sipped slowly, are effective. Chewing **Dill seeds** can help. If bad breath is caused by a disorder of the oral cavity, repeated gargling with 30 to 40 drops of **Myrrh tincture** diluted with lukewarm water is beneficial.

Wormwood tea is an excellent remedy for a **furred tongue** and **bad breath**. The saying: "Wormwood is beneficial and never does any harm" is not true. It should be used sparingly. Thence not quite half a teaspoon of Wormwood per cup is used.

BLADDER, weak

Many people suffer from a weak bladder, especially so on rainy days or when walking downhill. Warm **Yarrow and Horsetail sitz baths** – 100 gm. herbs per bath – are very beneficial (see General Information "sitz bath"). 4 cups of **Lady's Mantle tea** are to be drunk daily and the area of the bladder is rubbed with **Shepherd's Purse tincture** (see chapter "Shepherd's Purse") which tones up the muscles externally. Additionally **Shepherd's Purse** sitz baths are recommended (100 gm. herbs per bath). Excellent, too, are salt sitz baths. 1 handful of cooking salt is added to the warm sitz bath water. These sitz baths taken in the evening should be continued until the bladder functions normally.

CATARACT AND GLAUCOMA

Glaucoma is not only a disorder of the eye, rather it is caused by a malfunction of the kidneys. In most cases it occurs together with rheumatic pain in the joints. 2 to 3 cups of tea made from equal parts of **Stinging Nettle, Speedwell, Calendula and Horsetail** with a teaspoon of **Swedish Bitters** added to each cup should be drunk daily. Only freshly picked herbs should be used to speed up recovery.

For **cataract, Swedish Bitters** are brushed across the eyelids frequently. From letters I have received I can see that this treatment is effective (for exact details see chapter "Greater Celandine" page 25).

For glaucoma, **Horsetail sitz baths** are very important, since they relieve the pressure from the eyes, caused by a malfunction of the kidneys. These baths are so beneficial that the pressure is sometimes taken off the eyes during the bath. 100 gm. dried or about ½ bucketful of freshly picked herbs are soaked in cold water overnight; the water has to cover the herbs. The next day this is warmed and strained and the liquid is added to the bath water which should cover the kidney region but not the heart region. During the bath hot water is added to maintain an even temperature. Without drying and wrapped into a bathrobe, one should perspire for 1 hour in a pre-warmed bed.

STEAM BATH FOR THE EYES

20 gm. Eyebright 20 gm. Valerian 10 gm. Vervain 30 gm. Elder flowers 20 gm. Camomile	½ litre of white wine is brought to the boil and poured over 5 level tablespoons of these well-mixed herbs and the steam is allowed to penetrate the closed eyes. The wine is best stored in a bottle and, in small amounts, used to prepare further steam baths.

Cotton wool, moistened with Swedish Bitters, is applied to the closed eyes for 1 hour after lunch, to relieve the troublesome pain. – The eyes can be bathed with **Eyebright**, but the infusion has to be very weak. If the trouble worsens after this treatment, the infusion was too strong. Only half a teaspoon of Eyebright per cup is infused for a short time. I recommend compresses with this weak infusion applied to the eyes. The infusion has to be prepared fresh each time and should only be used once.

One day, after church, a woman, looking very happy, came up to me and said that her eyes had been affected by glaucoma and following the advice given in my book, her complaint disappeared.

CONSTIPATION

A physician once said during a talk he gave in a home for old people and which I attended: "The more you rely on laxatives, the more obstinate will your constipation become!" Besides, the intestines become weak through loss of fluid.

By taking 3 tablespoons of **Linseed** with a little liquid during each meal, digestion will become normal. **Figs and Prunes** soaked in cold water overnight, slightly warmed and eaten before or as a breakfast are also effective. If there is a natural well nearby, it is sufficient to drink 1 glass of this water on an empty stomach in the morning. Especially beneficial is **Wild Chicory** or Succory. Half a cup to one cup of this tea, drunk on an empty stomach, will increase the movements of the bowel and rid you of the most stubborn constipation.

I do not wish to withhold a letter I received from Bavaria: "Following your advice to drink **Chicory tea** and eat **Fig sausage**, my mother has now normal **bowel movements** after **20 years** of problems. She had already reconciled herself to the fact that nothing could help her."

Recipe for Fig sausage: ½ kilo of Figs, washed and minced, and 5 gm. of finely ground Senna leaves are kneaded and formed into sausages which are wrapped into aluminium foil and stored in the refrigerator. Every morning a piece, the size of a hazelnut (for children a third of this), is taken on an empty stomach, until normal bowel movements are achieved.

Another hint: Daily walking in the fresh air! More fruit, vegetables, bran and rye in the diet!

I would like to tell you how I came to know that **Chicory** is effective for **constipation**. My childhood is connected with memories of Chicory and its star-like flowers which grew along paths and were a very pleasant sight. Here, where I live now, I miss these blue flowers and very seldom do I find this plant. Therefore I was quite surprised, when, one day, I saw this plant growing across the road. I stopped, saying: "Despite your poor looks, I will pick your 6 flowers!" Now, every day, I made 6 cups of herb tea for my family and myself and the next day I added the 6 flowers. One flower ended in my cup. It so happened that this day I had a bowel movement after each meal; that makes 3 movements. It left me no peace until, in a very old herbal, I found the answer: Chicory is a very effective remedy in cases of obesity. With such copious but normal bowel movements I can imagine that gradually weight is lost!

DIABETES

Diabetes is on the increase and soon will be in front of all illnesses along with cardiac infarct and cancer. Our diet of too much and the wrong type of food is often the cause of this illness, especially in children. Yes, not only adults, but many children as well suffer from a **disorder of the pancreas** and are diabetic. It means a restriction in the pleasures of childhood, observing a strict diet and injecting insulin twice daily. Since many diseases of our time show that easy circumstances are not always good for us, we should tighten the belt and eat more wholesome food. Before holidays, people can be observed buying food, as if an army depended on it.

I would like to point out remedies which stimulate the pancreas and therefore take away the cause of diabetes. The **Swiss herbalist Abbé Kuenzle** says: "Diabetes is rather quickly remedied with tea made from the following herbs: 3 parts **Avens** (Geum alpina), 1 part **Blackberry leaves**, 1 part **Blueberry leaves**, 3 parts **Golden Fingergrass** (Potentilla aurea or Potentilla reptens) and 2 parts dried **green Beanpods**." 1 level teaspoon of this mixture is used for 1 cup of boiling water and infused for 3 minutes. Daily amount 1½ to 2½ litres.

The curative properties of **Blueberry leaves** depend on the time of gathering. They should only be **gathered before the fruit ripens**. When gathered at the right time, they are a clinically proven remedy for diabetes. Blueberry leaves, before the fruit ripen, contain Myrtillin which not only reduces the blood sugar but remedies the illness. The Myrtillin contained in the leaves is called, and rightly so, "vegetable insulin". Despite the excellent properties of Blueberry leaves, treatment with this tea should only be undertaken under medical supervision.

Celery reduces the blood sugar and is recommended. An old popular remedy is the raw **juice of "Sauerkraut"**, as well as the daily eating of raw **carrots**; also **onions and garlic** eaten on a piece of bread help to reduce the sugar level.

Another popular remedy: 4 tablespoons of **Blueberry leaves (picked before the berries ripen)** are added to 2 litres of cold water, brought to the boil and simmered until the water is reduced to half the amount. A cup of this decoction is taken 3 times a day. **Stinging Nettles**, too, have a favourable influence on the pancreas and reduce the blood sugar. In this case Stinging Nettle extract is used.

Since **Calamus root** remedies almost all disorders of the pancreas, it is beneficial for diabetes. 1 level teaspoon of Calamus roots are cold-soaked in a cup of water overnight, warmed slightly the next morning and strained. 1 sip of this infusion is taken before and after each meal; that makes 6 sips a day. These 6 sips alone will be felt beneficially by every diabetic.

Leaves and shoots of **Elder** are also recommended. Elder is one of our oldest medicinal herbs.

In early spring when **Dandelions** appear in meadows and fields, they can be used in salads, cut off near the roots and well washed. Dandelions with the yellowish juice taste better than ones with a greenish juice. Diabetics should eat Dandelion salad noon and evening every day in spring. When the Dandelions flower it is time to start a 4-week's treatment with the stems. They are picked with the flower still on, washed and only then the flower is removed. 10 to 15 stems are eaten every day and this treatment can reduce the sugar level in the blood effectively. At first the leaves have a somewhat bitter taste, but this improves.

Mistletoe as well influences the pancreas favourably. Mistletoe is cold-soaked overnight. In the beginning of this treatment 3 cups of water and 3 heaped teaspoons of Mistletoe are used. A few weeks later only 2 cups of water and 2 heaped teaspoons are used and again a few weeks later 1 cup and 1 heaped teaspoon is used. Then for a while this treatment is stopped altogether, when, come spring, fresh vegetables are available again. Mistletoe has curative properties from the beginning of October to the beginning of December and in the months of March and April and should be picked then.

Mistletoes growing on oaks and poplars are best, but also the ones growing on firs and fruit trees have curative properties. The stalks and leaves are cut. **The white berries are not to be used for infusions!**

Since our excellent **Swedish Bitters** influences the pancreas favourably, even remedies the disorder, it is also recommended. 1 teaspoonful in a little herb tea should be taken 3 times daily and externally it should be applied as a compress, left on for 4 hours, once a month.

Chicory roots are a wonderful dietary vegetable for diabetics. Since they taste rather bitter they are prepared with water similar to endive salad. Moreover a tea made from Chicory flowers and stems is used successfully to treat **obesity**; 2 cups are drunk daily.

The extracted juice of **Cucumbers** reduces the blood sugar and is therefore recommended.

Salsify is another excellent dietary vegetable, similar to **Asparagus**, and since its carbohydrate content is very low, it can be prepared with ample fat and breadcrumbs without causing harm.

Leeks are also excellent and a Leek salad for lunch is recommended. For the evening meal, Leeks, finely cut, are put on a piece of bread and eaten daily.

A tasty and easily digested drink is made of 500 gm. Leeks, finely cut to the top, macerated in 0.7 litre of dry **white wine** for 24 hours (the bottle is well stoppered), strained and bottled. A sip of this liquid is taken mornings and evenings. The residue can be eaten on a piece of bread.

A general practitioner helped a woman with the following recipe: 3 large cloves of **Garlic** are crushed and placed in a 1 litre bottle of rye whisky or wodka. This is left to stand in the sun or in a warm place for 10 to 14 days. 1 teaspoon of this liquid is taken before breakfast every day.

In April, 1977, I received a telephone call from Vienna and a woman who has had diabetes for 30 years asked me for help. I recommended the above mentioned applications of the various herbs.

She followed it exactly and at the beginning of August, I was told that a medical check-up had shown a normal sugar level. At the end of September I gave a talk in Vienna and this woman sought leave to speak and said: "For 30 years I was a diabetic. I followed Mrs. Treben's advice and since August I have a normal sugar level." She received thunderous applause.

An acquaintance from Bavaria wrote: "A good friend had **diabetes** for years and had to have injections of insulin daily. Now with the use of tea and herbs mentioned in your book his blood sugar has been reduced. Naturally he is constantly under medical supervision. His doctor was surprised about the lower sugar level."

An engineer from Vienna had a **sugar level** of 280. He followed the advice from this book and, during a medical check-up, it was found that the sugar count was 130.

Naturally the application of all these herbs and vegetables is only successful if the prescribed diet is strictly adhered to.

EMPHYSEMA

Emphysema, as well as **cardiac asthma and disorders of the thyroid gland**, with their shortness of breath, is caused largely through liver trouble. The upward pressure of the liver contributes to the swelling and enlargement of the bronchial tubes, lungs and the heart. The constant pressure on the sensitve thyroid gland causes abnormal changes. In such a case, 1 cup of **Common Club Moss tea** is drunk in the morning and **Swedish Bitters** is applied as a **compress** for 4 hours during the day (see chapter on Swedish Bitters "directions"). A **poultice of Horsetail** is applied overnight. 1 heaped handful of Horsetail is placed in a sieve and steamed over boiling water until it is soft and hot. Then, placed between a piece of linen, it is applied to the liver. The pressure is released and gradually the alarming shortness of breath eases.

ERYSIPELAS

The freshly picked leaves of **Coltsfoot** are washed and crushed to a pulp with a wooden rolling pin and applied to the inflamed areas. A decoction can be made from the leaves. The leaves are finely cut, boiling water is poured over them and infused for a short time and the decoction, cooled, applied as a compress.

Cabbage leaves, washed and crushed, can be used as well. Very soothing is the juice of the fleshy leaves of **Houseleek**; the leaves are put in the juice extractor and the juice is applied to the inflamed areas, or the leaves are cut lengthwise and placed on a plate with the cut area upward. The juice that seeps out is then applied to the inflamed area. In the morning, half an hour before breakfast, 1 cup of **Speedwell** tea is drunk and 3 to 4 cups of Stinging Nettle tea are sipped throughout the day until a medical check-up shows absence of erysipelas.

EYES, weeping

For this troublesome condition 10 gm. **Eyebright**, 10 gm. **Valerian**, 15 gm. **Avens** (Geum urbanum), 10 gm. **Lilac blossoms**, 15 gm. **Lady's Mantle**, 20 gm. **Camomile** and 10 gm. **Rue** are mixed. 15 gm. of this herb mixture are steeped in ½ litre of cold water overnight and the next morning brought to the boil, stirred, taken off the hotplate and infused for 3 minutes. When somewhat cooled, a piece of linen is soaked in the infusion and, still warm, applied to the closed eyes. This is repeated several times for half an hour. Afterwards a dry cloth is applied and the eyes are rested for a while.

FACIAL NEURALGIA

The flowers of the **Camomile, Yarrow, Mullein and Thyme**, picked in the sun, are put into a linen bag in their fresh state or lightly dried and this bag is applied to the aching areas. Only herbs that are picked in the sun are used, as their volatile oils are better developed. Additionally 4 cups of tea made of the mentioned herbs are sipped throughout the day. Should spasmodic pain develop, the face is washed with a warm decoction of **Stinging Nettle** and rubbed with a towel, then a linen bag filled with small cut **Common Club Moss** is applied. — Compresses made with **Swedish Bitters** (see page 52) must be applied while lying in bed. 1 teaspoon of Swedish Bitters diluted with the above mentioned tea mixture also brings relief.

FISTULAS

1 teaspoon, in bad cases 1 tablespoon, of **Swedish Bitters** in unsweetened **Camomile tea** is drunk three times daily. Externally, washings with a lukewarm decoction made from equal proportions of **Ground Ivy, Horsetail and Toadflax** (Linaria vulgaris) are undertaken. Afterwards the fistulas are dabbed with **Swedish Bitters**, or a piece of cotton wool moistened with Swedish Bitters, is applied. **Horsetail sitz baths** should be taken and **Horsetail poultices** should be applied (see chapter on Horsetail "directions").

GALL STONES

Interestingly more women than men have gall stones. Nausea, vomiting and agonizing pain which shoots up and across the right rib cage towards the heart are the symptoms. Since there are so many remedies available in God's Pharmacy, it does not always have to end in an operation.

A 6-week course treatment with **Radish juice** has helped every time, unless the stones are of the rare kind that do not dissolve. In this case an operation is necessary. Radishes are put in the juice extractor. To start with, 100 gm. are used and this is increased gradually to 400 gm. in 3 weeks and decreased gradually to 100 gm. in the following 3 weeks. Radish juice should not be taken if the lining of the stomach or the intestines are inflamed. How quickly gall stones are dissolved is illustrated by the following story: The wife of a retired general had her gall stones removed by an operation. She had kept the stones, varying in size and for fun had them mounted in the handle of a knife. One day while peeling radishes visitors arrived and she put the knife into the bowl with the radishes. When she returned after a time, the gall stones in the handle of the knife were dissolved in the radish pulp.

A herbal mixture of 20 gm. each of **Lesser Burnet, Ivy, Hops, Agrimony, Peppermint and Wormwood** is beneficial for colic and stones. 3 tablespoonfuls of this mixture are put into 1 litre of apple wine or cider, this is brought just to the boil, taken off the hot plate and infused for 3 minutes. 1 tablespoon of this liquid is taken every hour throughout the day, about 8 to 9 times. Since it should be taken warm, it is kept in a thermos flask.

GOITRE

Frequent gargling with a tea made from finely cut leaves of **Knotted Figwort** (Scrophularia nodosa) or **Bedstraw** will make a goitre disappear. Knotted Figwort grows in moist ditches, damp woods and on the side of brooks. It has insignificant reddish brown flowers and dark green pointed leaves. These have the same sharp smell as Elder leaves and are therefore not easily mistaken for another plant. Whereas only the leaves of Figwort are used to make a gargle which is not swallowed, the whole plant of Bedstraw is used and while gargling, some of it is swallowed from time to time. An acquaintance from Vienna developed a goitre in February, 1979. She was afraid of an operation and following my advice she started gargling with warm Bedstraw tea as soon as the first plants appeared in spring. A year later she was a happy woman and told me that her husband had gathered Bedstraw frequently and from the beginning she felt how the goitre decreased until there was no sign of it.

HAEMOPHILIA (HEMOPHILIA)

For this fortunately rare disease, the following herbs are used successfully: **Speedwell, Lady's Mantle, Shepherd's Purse, Yarrow and Horsetail** mixed in equal proportions. 1 heaped teaspoon per cup of boiling water is used and infused for 1 minute. At least 4 cups have to be drunk throughout the day. Besides this, sitz baths are taken with these herbs for 14 days. 100 gm. herbs are steeped in cold water overnight. The next day this is warmed up and the liquid is added to the warm sitz bath water. The bath should last for 20 minutes. The bath water can be poured back over the herbs and, warmed, re-used twice.

HAIR, beautiful

A handful each of freshly picked **Stinging Nettle, Walnut, Birch and Elder leaves** and 1 stem of **Greater Celandine** is put into cold water and brought to the boil, then infused for 3 minutes. With half of this decoction and pure soap the hair is washed thoroughly, then rinsed with clear water. The other half of the decoction is poured over the hair and left to penetrate for a few minutes, then the hair is dried without rinsing.

HAY FEVER

Since **Stinging Nettle** is beneficial for all cases of **allergy**, 3 to 4 cups of Stinging Nettle tea with three teaspoons of **Swedish Bitters** diluted with the tea, will bring relief in a relatively short time.

HEARING DISORDERS caused by colds

Ground Ivy, Sage and Yarrow are mixed in equal proportions. A warm infusion made of these herbs is used to rinse the ears. **Swedish Bitters** on a piece of cotton wool put into the ear, into which a few drops of warm **Thyme oil** have been poured first, is recommended, too. Thyme oil is warmed by placing a teaspoon in hot water and then putting 1 to 2 drops of oil on the spoon.

HEART AND CIRCULATION DISORDERS

Since **cardiac infarct** has increased much in the last years, I would like to point out a tea mixture which has shown surprising results **in heart and circulation disorders**.

10 gm. Dandelion	30 gm. Hawthorn	10 gm. Calamus	10 gm. Irish Moss (not Iceland M.)
20 gm. Mistletoe	10 gm. Knotgrass	10 gm. Rue	10 gm. Shepherd's Purse
20 gm. Yerba Mate	10 gm. Hemp Nettle	10 gm. Arnica	10 gm. Lesser Burnet
10 gm. Silverweed	10 gm. Fumitory	10 gm. Yarrow	10 gm. Rest-Harrow
10 gm. Motherwort	10 gm. Couch grass	10 gm. Burdock	10 gm. Bladder Wrack
10 gm. Beanpods	10 gm. Balm Mint	10 gm. Horsetail	10 gm. Frangula Bark

These herbs are mixed well and 1 heaped teaspoon per cup is used, steeped in cold water overnight and slightly heated the next morning. A cup of this tea sweetened with a teaspoonful of honey is drunk daily mornings and evenings.

HICCUPS

A tea made from **Dill seeds**, unsweetened, is a pleasant and swift acting remedy for hiccups. 1 teaspoon of Dill seeds per cup of boiling water is used and infused for 3 minutes.

KIDNEYS = GRAVEL IN THE BLADDER, KIDNEY STONES

A homoeopathic remedy is **Stinging Nettle essence** which can be recommended. It is available at special chemists' and health food stores. As mentioned in the chapter "Horsetail", **Horsetail sitz baths** during which **Horsetail tea** should be drunk, help to expel gravel from the kidneys and the bladder, as well as kidney stones. Old herbals mention **Crane's Bill** (Germanium robertanium), **Sweet Violet and Bearberry** (Urva ursi) as an effective and safe remedy for kidney stones. Bearberry's high tannin content is not always well tolerated and vomiting, nausea and loss of appetite may occur. Pear leaves can be used instead.

The yellow flowers of **Agrimony** whch grow along paths and fields, on slopes, on edges of woodland and waste ground make an excellent tea which effectively expels gravel and stones from the kidneys, as well as gall stones. A tea made from 20 gm. each of **Birch leaves, Agrimony, Rest-harrow and Shepherd's Purse** is most beneficial.

MENSTRUATION

For excessive menstrual flow 1 cup of tea made of the following herbs is drunk on an empty stomach half an hour before breakfast: 25 gm. **Arnica flowers**, 50 gm. **Valerian roots**, 25 gm. **Iceland Moss**, 25 gm. **Balm Mint**, 25 gm. **Yarrow** and 25 gm. **Sage**. 1 heaped teaspoon of this mixture per cup of boiling water is used, and this is infused for 3 minutes. Drinking this tea should be continued after the menstrual flow has become normal. These herbs have a very beneficial effect on the female organs which lasts for years. During **menopause** no unpleasant symptoms develop.

Years ago a young woman asked me for the recipe of this tea. Her menstrual flow was very heavy and she had had 2 treatments without success at the clinic of her brother who was a gynaecologist. The tea helped her condition as quickly as in my case, when after typhoid fever I suffered from heavy bleedings which would not stop. The doctor who attended me at that time throught we might now try herbs and that is how I came by this recipe. For more than 1½ years I had monthly bleedings which lasted up to 14 days and sometimes longer. 4 weeks after drinking this herb tea I had a normal menstrual flow. I continued to drink this tea for 5 years.

MISCARRIAGES

Many women suffer from recurrent miscarriages; they cannot carry the baby for the full term. These women should drink Yarrow and Lady's Mantle tea, 2 to 3 cups daily. But also young shoots of **Hornbeams** which are planted as a living fence around houses bring relief. The young leaf tops consisting of 3 leaves are boiled in milk which is then strained, one egg yolk is beaten into it and a white sauce is added. This soup should be eaten as an evening meal for several weeks, even months. A miscarriage will hardly occur anymore.

MULTIPLE SCLEROSIS

For this, described as an incurable illness, help can be found in God's Pharmacy. It might be a very slow process but do not give up and lose hope and faith in the herbs which our Creator has given to sick mankind. I want to point out that only freshly picked herbs should be used for serious diseases.

Shepherd's Purse is washed, finely cut and put into a bottle up to the neck. 38% to 40% rye whisky or wodka is poured over it and left to stand in the sun or near the stove for 10 days. The affected parts of the muscles are rubbed 2 to 3 times a day. 4 cups of **Lady's Mantle tea** and 2 cups of **Sage tea** are sipped throughout the day. The freshly picked leaves of **Wood Sorrel** are washed and still wet put into the juice extractor. This juice is taken in 3 to 5 drop doses diluted with tea every hour for six hours every day. Rubs or massages with **St. John's Wort, Camomile and Thyme oil** (see respective chapters "directions") are also beneficial.

Flowers of **St. John's Wort, Camomile and Yarrow** are macerated like Shepherd's Purse. These tinctures are rubbed on the spine, joints and the hips. Also recommended are massages with **Comfrey tincture**. Comfrey roots are washed, cut and macerated in alcohol (40% content). If there is stiffness in the spine, **Comfrey meal** as a poultice is applied. This meal is made into a paste with hot water and a few drops of oil are added to make it more spreadable. 1 cup of **Yarrow tea** is drunk in the morning and one in the evening and 3 tablespoons of Swedish Bitters diluted with herb tea are sipped throughout the day. Compresses with **Swedish Bitters** should also be applied repeatedly to the back of the head for 4 hours.

Sitz baths made from **Pine sprigs, St. John's Wort, Camomile, Sage, Yarrow, Thyme and Horsetail** should not be forgotten, since all these herbs have a beneficial effect on paralysis. 100 gm. of herbs per bath are used, steeped in cold water overnight. This is warmed the next day and the liquid added to the bath water which should cover the kidney region.

The baths should last for 20 minutes and 1 hour should be spent in bed perspiring. This bath water can be re-used twice by pouring it again over the herbs and warming it. Each week only 1 sort of herb should be used.

Especially recommended are **Thyme baths** which influence the muscles and the tissue, but also **Stinging Nettle baths** which stimulate the blood supply should not be forgotten: For these, 200 gm. of herbs per bath are used and prepared like sitz baths and the bath water can be re-used 3 times. The heart region has to stay outside the water.

Cow-parsnip poultices applied to the whole body give good results. The leaves are washed, crushed to a pulp with a wooden rolling pin and spread on to a sheet. This and a bath towel are wrapped around the patient and left on overnight. If he feels a drawing and nervous pain in very sensitive parts, he must be unwrapped. Mostly he will feel the beneficial effect of the herbs and sleep well. Often there is a noticeable improvement. At the same time I would like to point out that a change of diet has also had notable results.

A special remedy for this illness could be **mare's milk**. Since horse-breeding is on the increase it might be possible to get such milk. An acquaintance told me, years ago she read that an old shepherd cured several illnesses which were considered incurable with this milk.

The following is an account of a woman who has **multiple sclerosis** and also suffers from **bladder and abdominal trouble**: "I have followed your suggestion to rub the back with Yarrow tincture in the evening and the legs with Shepherd's Purse tincture mornings and evenings, as well as to apply Swedish Bitters as a compress on the abdomen, daily. I also drink Willow-herb tea with Swedish Bitters on an empty stomach half an hour before breakfast. Now, 4 months later, I can say that your advice is very good and that the herb treatment is starting to have an effect. The terrible, painful cramps in the legs are slowly easing and are less painful. Some days I am able to make a few steps without holding onto anything. My bladder functions normally again. I have menstrual periods every 3 to 5 weeks, but now they only last 3 to 5 days. This is a success for me, even if still small. Multiple sclerosis is a very stubborn disease with many side effects. Daily I take a small amount of Swedish Bitters in Stinging Nettle, Yarrow and Lady's Mantle tea. I have also had good results with Greater Celandine. For years I have had a thick **scab** below the left **eye** which grew closer to the eye with time. I tried several kinds of medication without results and have now tried Greater Celandine juice (Greater Celandine macerated in rye whisky or wodka for 10 days). The scab has almost disappeared. I am so pleased about each little result which incites me to keep going. I have supplied myself with enough herbs for winter."

Because I suffered from **disc lesions** I looked through a medical book that belonged to my parents and read: Grind **Peony** roots and bathe in the decoction. Peonies are beneficial to the brain and the spinal cord. I made 2 baths from them, I macerated the roots in rye whisky or wodka and added some of the tincture to the decoction in which I bathed for 20 minutes. The next day the pain was gone. Since then 3 weeks have passed and the pain has not recurred.

During a talk I gave in Rendsburg, West Germany, a lady walked onto the platform and told that, 3 years ago, she had been confined to a wheelchair. By following all suggestions in "God's Pharmacy" her condition improved so far that today she is able to walk normally and feels a healthy person. She had bought all the herbs she needed dried, since there was no opportunity to gather fresh herbs. The audience showed appreciation by applauding her, for having had the strength to start and to keep up the treatment.

Mongoloid, spastic or handicapped children are treated with the same herbs that are used for multiple sclerosis and muscular atrophy. Massages with the mentioned tinctures and especially the invigorating herb baths cannot be recommended enough. In many cases some of the causes lie within the mother's behaviour during pregnancy. Besides cigarettes, alcohol and drugs, coffee should be avoided.

Children with **speech disorders** should have this treatment too. In all 4 cases compresses with Swedish Bitters (see chapter "Swedish Bitters") applied to the back of the head are important.

MUSCULAR ATROPHY

For this illness the following herb treatment has been proved beneficial: Freshly picked **Shepherd's Purse** is washed, finely cut and put into a bottle. 38% to 40% rye whisky or wodka is poured over it and this is left to stand in the sun or near the stove for 10 days. Then some of the liquid is poured into a small bottle for use and some more alcohol is added to the large bottle.

The affected muscles are massaged with this tincture 3 times daily and 4 cups of **Lady's Mantle tea** are sipped throughout the day; if possible only freshly picked herbs should be used (see chapters "Shepherd's Purse" and "Lady's Mantle").

NAILBED, infection of the — NAILS, injured or brittle

For infection of the nailbed 50 gm. of **Mallow** are steeped in cold water overnight; before going to bed, hands or feet are bathed in this cold infusion, slightly warmed, for 20 minutes. This infusion, kept cold, can be re-used 2 or 3 times. Calendula ointment is smeared on the infected nailbed and then a Swedish Bitters compress is applied.

Brittle or injured nails are brushed with **Onion or Crowfoot juice** (Ranunculus). An Onion is halved and rubbed onto the nail or put in the juice extractor and the juice applied. The round stem of the **Crowfoot** is opened and the juice applied to the nail. This has to be done frequently, a once-only application does not give results.

NIGHT SWEATS

Through the ages, **Sage** has been esteemed as a good remedy for night sweats. A tea is made and drunk on an empty stomach each morning for a prolonged period. This treatment rids the body of the substances which are the cause of night sweats: A reliable remedy found in old herbals is the following mixture: 20 gm. each of **Sage, Lady's Mantle and Horsetail**. This is infused for a short time and 1 cup is drunk before breakfast. These herbs strengthen the body and rid it of night sweats.

The last time I was at a Kneipp Spa, an old lady told me that she suffered from night sweats — was there anything she could do? I recommended Sage tea, 1 cup before going to bed. A few days later I met her on a walk: She could hardly believe it but after drinking Sage tea for 4 days she no longer suffered from night sweats: "But I have the feeling", she said smilingly, "that you know how **quickly the herbs give relief.**"

OEDEMA (EDEMA) or SWELLINGS caused by retention of fluid in the tissues

Two teaspoons of finely cut **Rest-harrow** roots per cup of cold water are steeped overnight, warmed slightly in the morning and strained. Half a cup is drunk half an hour before and the other half cup half an hour after breakfast.

A second possibility is to treat Edema with **Elder bark** or twigs. 1 teaspoon, just level, of **Elder bark** (a larger amount could cause diarrhoea or vomiting) is steeped in a cup of cold water overnight. To make it weaker half a cup of water can be added, warmed slightly and half a cup of this is drunk after each of the 3 meals.

PHIMOSIS

A method used by Dr. Dirk Arntzen or Berlin is to treat Phimosis in children (it does not work with older men) with baths. 10 to 12 ml. of a freshly prepared 10% **potassium sulphate solution** are used for the child's warm bath, about 50 to 75 litres. Sometimes after 3 to 4 baths, results are obtained, surprisingly also in extreme cases. Hence many children would not need an operation.

Mallow baths show results, too. 1 handful of Mallow per bath is steeped in cold water overnight. For adults 100 gm. herbs per sitz bath are used.

PROLAPSE OF THE UTERUS

4 cups of **Lady's Mantle tea** are sipped throughout the day. 1 heaped teaspoon of herbs per cup of boiling water is infused for a short time. A bottle is filled up to the neck with finely cut **Shepherd's Purse**, stems, leaves and flowers, 38% to 40% rye whisky or wodka is poured in and the bottle is left to stand in the sun or near the stove for 10 days.

Several times a day the left side of the abdomen from the vagina upward is massaged with this tincture. As well, 3 **Yarrow sitz baths** a week are taken: 100 gm. Yarrow are steeped in cold water overnight, heated the next day and used in the sitz bath which should last for 20 minutes. The bath water is poured back over the herbs twice so that it can be used for 3 baths.

PSORIASIS

There are several kinds of this disorder, in some cases the skin affected is **bright red and sharply defined**, in another the skin is covered in **scales** and the third kind has **thick leathery, cracked skin**. These cracks deepen and open up towards the evening and cause the people affected great pain. On top of this the intense itching is very troublesome. The skin sheds a great amount of scales daily and every movement causes showers of scales.

Years ago, I heard of a 38 year old woman whose skin from the neck downward was cracked and leathery. Her hair had fallen out and she was in a miserable state. At the hospital she was put up to her neck into a plastic bag. The skin became softer and was therefore less painful, but her condition could not be remedied. At that time I realized that only diet and herbs that purify the blood, ridding it of toxic substances, could heal this condition. When this woman drank the tea recommended by me and followed the appropriate diet her condition improved within 6 months. Her hair grew again and her skin became smooth and showed no patches. Since then I have been able to help many people who suffered from this condition.

This skin disorder is caused by a **malfunction of the liver** and therefore, besides herbs, a liver diet should be adhered to: Sausages, pork and smoked meat as well as soups should be avoided, acid foods and drinks such as orange, lemon, grapefruit, wine, cider, vinegar, berries, as well as black current, and their juices are included in this. Fresh apples, coffee, cocoa, chocolate and honey, since these latter form acids which the liver cannot tolerate, as well as all kinds of tinned fish, smoked fish, tinned meat, vegetables like beans, peas, lentils and alcohol in any form are also not allowed. Permitted are milk foods, milk and milk products, salads prepared with sour cream, veal, chicken, boiled beef, venison, fresh or frozen fish, some vegetables and, as a substitute for fresh fruit, lots of stewed apples should be eaten.

Tea mixture:	30 gm. Willow bark	10 gm. Oak bark
	40 gm. Goat's Beard	30 gm. Speedwell
	30 gm. Greater Celandine	20 gm. Fumitory
	50 gm. Stinging Nettle	30 gm. Calendula
	20 gm. Walnut husks	20 gm. Yarrow

1 heaped teaspoonful of this mixture per cup of boiling water is used and infused for 3 minutes. If possible freshly picked herbs should be used. 1½ to 2 litres of this tea are sipped throughout the day. Each sip is immediately taken up by the body and used.

Twice a day lard has to be applied to the skin. Should the body be covered in scabs, an ointment, made from Greater Celandine juice (the plant is put into the juice extractor), 5 gm. of juice per 50 gm. of lard, is applied. This ointment is stored in the refrigerator. Freshly pressed juice of Mallow could be used to prepare an ointment, as well.

Recommended are baths made from an infusion of **Crane's Bill** (Geranium robertanium). Mallow and Horsetail baths (both herbs are used in equal proportions, steeped in cold water overnight − 200 gm. of herbs per bath − the bath should last for 20 minutes and the heart region has to be outside the water) relieve the itching and promote healing. All these applications are also beneficial for **neurodermatitis**.

2 children of the same family suffered from psoriasis, the 12 year old girl, since she had been 2 years old, the boy for 9 months. The parents had consulted many doctors and tried everything, without result. The herbs which the children had enjoyed gathering in the summer, remedied this condition. The mother told me that now the girl has a skin as smooth as a baby's. She continues to drink small amounts of the tea.

In another case a 12 year old girl had her face covered in red patches since she was two years old. Her desperate parents had tried everything. 4 months after starting to drink the tea made from my recipe the girl had normal facial skin.

A business woman from Upper Austria had many areas of her skin affected by this disorder. Following my advice she used the above mentioned treatment and 4 weeks later improvement showed. The red patches gradually disappeared. In a similar case involving a miller who lives near Mainz, Germany, the red patches disappeared in a short time after he had started the treatment.

A nun who had suffered from this skin disorder for 30 years started the diet and drinking the tea at the beginning of October. At Christmas she told me that the scales had disappeared.

In October 1972 I learned that a young woman, mother of 3 children, suffered from this terrible skin disorder. It had developed after a case of jaundice and I assumed it was caused by an impaired liver function. The woman was completely covered in scales, even her scalp was affected. Her hair fell out until she was forced to wear a wig. Every movement resulted in showers of "dandruff". In the evening deep cracks formed. This woman, used to staying up till midnight sewing for her children and helping her husband in his business during the day, was now hardly able to stay up until 8 p.m. and had to go to bed wrapped in a sheet. Now and then she spent several weeks in hospital where she was put into a plastic bag up to her neck which softened the skin. The tea made from the above mentioned blood purifying herbs, together with the diet, remedied her disorder in 6 months. Already at the beginning of December she was less exhausted and tired. At Easter the following year her skin was smooth and her hair thick and beautiful.

A letter from Munich: In September 1977 I had asked your advice for my then 13 year old son Martin. The doctor's diagnosis was: **Neurodermatitis**. For 13 years we have been consulting pediatricians, dermatologists and naturopaths without results. The doctors prescribed cortisone again and again. When 7 years old, Martin stayed in Davos for 2 months. The doctor there told us that the disorder was inherited and there was no cure for it. It should be treated with cortisone. What followed in the weeks and years after his stay there was terrible. Bouts of fever, festering sores on the soles of his feet up to the ankles, on his palms, the back of his knee, also open sores developed on his earlobes, neck and face. The worst was the itching and the swollen glands in the groin which made walking very painful. After an intense treatment with cortisone appendicitis developed. At that time the doctor told us: "Be glad that it was appendicitis, other children develop stomach ulcers after this treatment." Tests showed that Martin was allergic to grass, hair, pollen, fungi and dust. From February 1973 to July 1978 a desensitizing course was given, but no improvement showed. Since 1977 Martin drinks about 1½ litres of the tea per day for psoriasis according to your recommendation. In the beginning he drank it only very reluctantly, it did not surprise us, as he had tried so many things without result. He had lost hope. Then he observed an increase in the amount of water he passed. 2 weeks later, when I came into his room to wake him up in the morning, he told me: "Mummy, I was hardly in bed and I fell asleep!" Going to bed for him was − one can say since he was a baby − a nightmare. Between the itching and the scratching he could not go to sleep and lay awake for hours. From then on Martin was convinced that the tea was effective and he tried to drink the prescribed quantity. The condition of his skin has improved quite a bit. He still scratches, but since drinking this tea no infection has developed. We can hardly believe it. Since January 1978 he is without bandages and cotton gloves. Martin is in High school and 1977/78 was the first year when he was not sick for weeks and months. You can imagine how happy he is and since September, after 4 years' absence, he is able to participate in sports. In July the course of desensitization was finished. The doctors at the hospital cannot explain the improvement of his skin disorder.

In the Summer of 1979 a specialist from West Germany came to see me with his 21 year old son who suffered from neurodermatitis since his birth. At first, when he started using the herbs, he developed strong reactions, such as pressure in the head and a blocked nose. Horsetail baths agreed with him, but he tolerated not as well the ones made from Crane's Bill, although the skin profited by them. Because his skin was very dry Hametum ointment to which freshly pressed Mallow juice had been added was applied. In this case, too, an improvement is noticeable, but above all the young man is sure he will be cured. In the middle of October 1979 he has taken up his law studies again.

RECEDING GUMS AND LOOSE TEETH

For this affliction the following herb mixture is recommended: **Knotgrass, Lady's Mantle, Oak bark and Sage** in equal proportions are steeped in cold water overnight. 2 heaped teaspoons per ½ litre are used. In the morning the tea is warmed slightly and kept in a thermos flask which has been rinsed with hot water. The mouth is rinsed repeatedly during the day with this tea. A toothbrush dipped in this tea can be used to massage the gums.

SCHOOL REPORT, poor (of children)

A desperate mother told me that her 12 year old son was totally disinterested at school; his teachers remarked that he did not follow the lessons and could not be motivated. The boy who was hardly ever sick before and used to enjoy sports now was pale and had rings under the eyes. To my mind he had to be ill. I recommended 2 cups of **Stinging Nettle tea** and 2 teaspoons of **Swedish Bitters** a day. In the short time of 6 weeks there were surprises on all sides, on the teacher's, the parent's and finally the boy's himself. The sudden good reports incited him to work harder and perform better at school.

SHAKING PALSY (PARKINSON'S DISEASE)

The freshly picked leaves of **Wood Sorrel** which cover the forest ground like a carpet are washed and put in the juice extractor. Every hour 3 to 5 drops of this juice are taken diluted with **Yarrow tea**. 4 to 5 cups of Yarrow tea are prepared every day, 1 heaped teaspoon of Yarrow flowers per cup. The dilution has to be at least 3 times the amount of the drops. At the same time the spine is rubbed with the freshly pressed juice of Wood Sorrel alternated with Yarrow tincture (see chapter on "Yarrow"). During the day **Swedish Bitters** is applied as a compress to the back of the head and left on for 4 hours (see chapter on "Swedish Bitters", page 52). − **Thyme baths** are taken, if stiffness in the limbs develops (200 gm. of **Thyme per bath**). This bath can be re-used twice if warmed up (see General Information "baths").

SHINGLES

The soothing **juice of Houseleeks** (Sempervivum tectorum) quickly relieves the deep pain caused by shingles. 4 to 5 fleshy leaves are cut lengthwise and placed on a plate. The juice, seeping to the surface, is applied to the affected areas several times a day. The leaves can also be put in the juice extractor. The sufferer feels the beneficial effects already after the first application. The following recipe is from an old herbal:

10 gm. Camomile 10 gm. Lady's Mantle 10 gm. Melilot 25 gm. Oak bark 20 gm. Oats 25 gm. Sage	Four tablespoons of these well-mixed herbs are put into one litre of cold water, brought just to the boil, taken off the hot-plate and infused for 3 minutes. The affected areas are gently dabbed with this lukewarm infusion several times a day. The warm herb residue, placed on a piece of linen, is applied overnight.

SLEEP, FITFUL (in children)

If children, during sleep, throw themselves from one side to the other and cannot find peace, a **Linden flower bath** has a soothing effect straight away. A large bucket is half filled with Linden flowers and cold water is poured over them. This is left to stand overnight, heated the next day, strained and the liquid is added to the bath water. The bath should last for 20 minutes. Rewarmed it can be used 2 more times. The Linden flowers should be picked as far as possible in bright sunshine.

SPINAL INJURIES

For this **Bedstraw ointment** is used most successfully. This ointment is prepared in the same way as Calendula ointment (see chapter on "Calendula") and is applied upward along the spine. Massages made with **Yarrow and Comfrey tincture** (see General Information "tinctures") are important as well as **Thyme** and **Yarrow baths** (see General Information "baths").

STRAWBERRY MARKS

The leaves of **Thuja** are washed, cut and placed in a bottle up to the neck, then 38% to 40% rye whisky or wodka is poured over them and this is left to stand in the sun or near the stove for 10 days. The strawberry mark is dabbed with this tincture several times a day.

The juice of **Houseleek leaves** (Sempervivum tectorum) which are cut lengthwise is brushed on the strawberry mark and gradually it will disappear. Fleshy **Calendula stems** are put in the juice extractor and the juice brushed on the mark is also beneficial. **Swedish Bitters**, used repeatedly, will also remove this condition. — The juices and tinctures mentioned can also be applied on **birthmarks, liver spots, brown and white patches and warts**.

A 2 year old boy had a strawberry mark the size of a lentil which was to be removed surgically. The anxious mother, afraid of complications, started to dab Swedish Bitters onto the mark repeatedly throughout the day. 6 weeks later the strawberry mark had disappeared.

STROKE (prophylactic measures)

Noticeable signs before a stroke are great restlessness, dizziness, anxiety, distorted face and hearing deceptions. A doctor should be consulted immediately! Above all eating moderately and taking slow walks are recommended. Alcohol (except Swedish Bitters), smoking and coffee are prohibited. **Mistletoe** prepared as a cold infusion, 1 cup in the morning and 1 cup in the evening, and 2 cups of **Sage tea** drunk throughout the day are recommended as well as **Swedish Bitters** applied as a compress to the heart region and moist cold compresses applied to the heart.

A tea made of the following herbs is recommended: **Angelica roots, Avens, Five-leaf Grass, Hyssop, Lavender flowers, Marjoram, Masterwort, Rosemary, Sage, Silverweed, Sweet Violet and Valerian roots**. These herbs are mixed well in equal proportions and then 1 cup of apple cider, heated just to the boiling point, is poured over 1 heaped teaspoon of herbs and infused for 3 minutes. This amount, prepared freshly several times a day and drunk, can prevent a stroke, when the above mentioned symptoms have been noticed.

STROKE (after a stroke with paralysis)

First of all a **Mistletoe course of treatment** should be applied. For 6 weeks, 3 cups, for 3 weeks, 2 cups and for 2 weeks, 1 cup of Mistletoe tea are drunk. 1 heaped teaspoon of Mistletoe per cup of cold water is steeped overnight, warmed the next morning and strained. The warm tea is kept in a thermos flask which has been rinsed with hot water.

1 heaped teaspoon of **St. John's Wort, Speedwell, Lavender, Balm, Rosemary and Sage**, mixed in equal proportions, is steeped in a cup (¼ litre) of boiling water for a short time. One cup of this tea is drunk during the morning and 1 cup during the afternoon.

Swedish Bitters applied as a **compress** to the back of the head stimulates the blood supply. The affected part of the body is massaged with **Yarrow, St. John's Wort, Shepherd's Purse or Thyme tincture. Thyme oil and St. John's Wort oil** used as a massage, are recommended, too. A bottle is filled up to the neck with the respective herbs. For the tinctures, 38% to 40% rye whisky or wodka spirit is poured in; for the herb oils, cold pressed olive oil is used. The herbs should be covered and left to stand in the sun or near the stove for 10 days.

In addition **Yarrow and Horsetail sitz baths**, 100 gm. of herbs per bath, are taken. The herbs are steeped overnight and heated the next morning. The liquid is added to the bath water. The baths should last for 20 minutes and the heart region has to be outside the water, when taking a full bath. The bath water can be re-used twice. For the bath one kind of herb should be used per week.

Warm **Comfrey leaf poultices** tone up the paralysed part. Hot water is poured over the leaves, these are then placed on a piece of linen and applied. – At night, the patient can put his head on a pillow filled with dried **Fern leaves** (the stems are removed). This is very beneficial.

Our granny, when 94 years old, had a slight stroke. When she awoke in the morning she could not speak and the left eyelid covered the eye halfway. Immediately we applied cold compresses on the forehead and the eyes. This was done 3 to 4 times as recommended by the Abbé Kneipp. When the doctor arrived she was allright again. She ate a light lunch still in bed, but in the evening she ate with us at the table.

TREMORS

For this disorder 50 gm. **St. John's Wort, 20 gm. Orchis, 20 gm. Cowslip and 10 gm. Juniper berries** are steeped in 38% to 40% rye or fruit spirit for 14 days. 15 to 20 drops of this tincture are taken hourly in the following herb tea of which 3 cups are drunk daily: 20 gm. each of **Ash leaves, Horsetail, Sage, St. John's Wort and Yarrow** are mixed well and 1 heaped teaspoon per cup of boiling water is used. Sitz baths made from **Pine needles, St. John's Wort, Thyme or Yarrow** are taken, 100 gm. of herbs per sitz bath. Since these sitz baths have a beneficial effect 3 sitz baths every 2 weeks are taken (see General Information "sitz baths").

WHITLOW

The affected finger should be bathed in a **Camomile infusion** for half an hour, several times a day. Afterwards an ointment for abscess is applied and then a clay pack. An old remedy mentions bathing the hand in milk in which **Garlic** had been boiled for half an hour. If the finger is festering, a poultice of **Linseed meal** is applied. Should the abscess break, the finger is bathed in a warm Camomile infusion and a compress with St. John's Wort oil is applied.

Another household remedy: **Elder flowers, Fern roots, Lesser Burnet, and Marsh Mallow** are used in equal proportions and 15 gm. of this mixture are steeped in ½ litre of **white wine** overnight and brought to the boil the next morning. The finger is bathed in this herb wine for 2 hours, then chalk powder is applied and the finger is bandaged.

WORMS

Pumpkin seeds are a traditional remedy for worms. For **threadworms** children are given 10 to 15 seeds a day and adults 20 to 30 seeds. The seeds, with the skin left on, should be chewed slowly and 1 hour later 1 level teaspoon of castor oil is taken.

For **tapeworms** Pumpkin seeds are recommended, too. While following a strict diet, 80 to 100 seeds (the thin skin is left on!), in 4 portions, are chewed well and 1 hour later half a tablespoon of castor oil is taken. If this treatment shows no result, it can be repeated without causing any harmful side effects.

An old remedy for **maw worms is carrot and beetroot**. The raw juice of **sauerkraut** is effective in expelling worms and the eating of **horseradish and onions**, as well as **garlic boiled in milk**, is also beneficial.

***

ADVICE FOR MALIGNANT DISEASES

Diseases of the BONE

4 cups of **Yarrow tea** are drunk daily, since Yarrow beneficially affects the production of healthy blood cells in the bone marrow. Additionally 2 cups of **Calendula tea** and 2 cups of **Stinging Nettle tea** are drunk to **purify the blood** (if possible use herbs in their fresh state and 1 heaped teaspoon per cup of water). 1 tablespoon of **Swedish Bitters** is added to 1 cup of tea and half this amount is drunk half an hour before and half an hour after each meal. **Yarrow tincture and Swedish Bitters** are used as a friction several times a day and so is **Comfrey tincture** (see "directions" under respective headings). If there is a tumour on the bone, the treatment mentioned under the heading "tumours" is applied. Should the pain in the bone be caused by **metastasis**, the area from which they originate has to be treated.

Diseases of the BREAST

Treatment commences after an operation. **Calendula ointment** is applied to the scars up to under the arm (see chapter on "Calendula"). Slightly warmed, the Calendula residues can be applied 4 to 5 times. This helps to smooth the skin and to give it back its normal colour; it relieves the drawing pain caused by the contraction of the scar tissue. If the lymph glands are affected, freshly picked **Plantain leaves** (Ribwort or Common Plantain) are applied as a poultice the same way as described in "lymph glands".

300 gm. **Calendula**, 100 gm. **Yarrow** and 100 gm. **Stinging Nettle** are mixed well and 1 heaped teaspoon per cup of boiling water is used. 1½ to 2 litres of this tea should be sipped throughout the day. 3 times a day, 1 tablespoon of **Swedish Bitters** is added to ½ cup of this tea and half this amount is sipped half an hour before and half an hour after each meal.

If there is pain, **Swedish Bitters as a compress and Horsetail as a poultice** are applied (see "General Information"). The mentioned treatments are also applied, if new lumps develop. Since the breasts and the reproductive organs are closely connected, the treatment under the heading "ovaries and uterus" should be noted and applied.

A young woman reports: "2 weeks after the birth of my child I noted **hard lumps** in my breast and the **nipple** became **infected**. It was very painful and I ran a fever. **Swedish Bitters**, applied as a compress overnight, brought immediate relief. – I have a farm and one day I noticed one cow's udder inflamed and hardened. Figuring that, if Swedish Bitters is used effectively on humans, animals, too, might profit. I tried the treatment and was pleasantly surprised by the result obtained within a short time."

Diseases of the INTESTINES

1 level teaspoon of **Calamus roots** is cold-soaked overnight, warmed the next morning and strained. 1 sip of this tea is taken shortly before and after each meal – that makes 6 sips a day – more should not be taken!

Additionally the following herb mixture is needed: 200 gm. **Calendula**, 100 gm. **Stinging Nettle** and 100 gm. **Yarrow**. 1 heaped teaspoon of these well-mixed herbs per cup of boiling water is used. The amount of tea needed per day is 1½ to 2 litres and it can be kept in a thermos flask. The patient takes a sip every quarter of an hour or every 20 minutes. This way the tea is easily digested. Experience has shown that, by drinking this tea, appetite will return.

In addition, 3 times a day, 1 tablespoon of Swedish Bitters is added to half a cup of this tea and half the amount is drunk half an hour before and the other half, half an hour after each meal. Should the amount of Swedish Bitters not be tolerated, 1 teaspoon instead of 1 tablespoon is used.

Besides, **Swedish Bitters as a compress** is applied to the entire abdomen. A large piece of cotton wool is moistened with Swedish Bitters and thinly spread over the abdomen. **Horsetail poultices** ease the pain and are applied as often as possible, perhaps for 2 hours mornings and afternoons, later overnight (see General Information "Swedish Bitters and poultices").

On October 1st, 1979, a couple, Helmut and Berta E. from Hamburg, came to my place to thank me for the help they had received from my book "Health through God's Pharmacy". Mrs. Berta E., now 53 years old, developed a very painful **pelvic tumour** after falling down the stairs. She underwent an operation in January 1977 and the diagnosis was: The tumor cannot be removed, because of too many growths. 7 weeks later she was discharged, her hair had fallen out and she knew she had cancer. In November 1978 she was again admitted to the same hospital for another operation and a 7 week treatment on the right side of the abdomen. During a post treatment in February 1979 a cyst the size of a child's head was found in the left side of the abdomen. In March 1979 she underwent another operation and **secondary growths** had already developed. For five weeks she was fed intravenously as she could not keep down any food.

At this time her husband was told by the doctors who attended her that her condition was hopeless. Her weight had dropped from 80 to 62 kilos. Just then Mr. E. was given a copy of my book "Health through God's Pharmacy". He bought the required herbs, Calendula, Stinging Nettle and Yarrow, as well as Calamus roots and several litres of Swedish Bitters at a chemist's in Hamburg. With the permission of the hospital's doctors, Swedish Bitters as a compress was applied over the entire abdomen as described in the book, and Mrs. E. drank the herb teas and took the 6 sips of Calamus root tea.

Within 48 hours, after continuous treatment, a hardly expected change in Mrs. E.'s condition occurred which astonished the medical personnel and all persons concerned. 10 days later on April 24th, 1979, Mrs. E. was discharged in "relatively good health", as medically quoted, for further treatment as an out-patient. She was so weak that for weeks she had to rest in bed. The treatment with the herbs and tea was continued conscientiously. Her general condition improved week by week. Her appetite returned and her weight increased gradually. Mr. Helmut E. said in a letter of August 8th, 1979 that this "miracle" could only have happened through God's blessing. Many of his friends, acquaintances and relatives have now turned to herbs. Towards the end of his letter he wrote: "My wife and I authorize explicitly the publication of 'our case', thus to give hope to people in need."

Diseases of the KIDNEYS

In this case, 4 cups a day are sipped of the following herb tea which the Swiss herbalist Abbé Kuenzle recommends for **cirrhosis** of the kidneys: **Golden Rod, Bedstraw and Yellow Dead Nettle** in equal proportions. To 3 cups of this tea 1 teaspoon of **Swedish Bitters** is added.

Horsetail sitz baths, lasting 20 minutes, are taken. 100 gm. of herbs per bath, are cold-soaked overnight, heated in the morning, strained and the liquid added to the bath water. Then the bath water is poured back over the herbs, so that 3 sitz baths can be made from the one lot of herbs. Warm **Horsetail poultices** are applied overnight and **Swedish Bitters as compresses** is applied to the kidney region for 4 hours during the day.

Diseases of the LARYNX

Mallow loses one third of its medicinal properties during the drying process, therefore it is essential to use only fresh plants. 1 heaped teaspoon per cup is used and 2½ litres of tea are needed daily. The herbs are steeped in cold water overnight, warmed slightly the next morning and strained. The tea is kept warm in a thermos flask which has been rinsed with hot water, or the required amount is re-warmed in a water-bath. 4 cups of this tea are taken in **sips** and 6 cups are used for **rinsing and gargling**.

These 10 cups bring about the abatement of the existing malignant disease of the larynx very soon, even when the disease is advanced. The residue from the daily tea preparation is left in the pot, in the evening re-warmed with a little water, mixed with **barley flour** (available from health food stores) and warmed again. This poultice is spread on a piece of linen and applied to the larynx. A warm cloth is wrapped around. After the first application the person will feel a marked relief and often, 4 to 5 days later, he regains his voice.

This same treatment is used for a **disorder of the oesophagus (esophagus)**. Besides the warm Barley meal poultices, warm Horsetail poultices are applied overnight (see "General Information" and "Horsetail") deep gargling with fresh **Bedstraw tea** is also recommended (see "tongue").

LEUKAEMIA (LEUKEMIA)

Tea mixture:	20 gm. Wormwood	30 gm. Stinging Nettle
20 gm. Speedwell	30 gm. Elder shoots	15 gm. St. John's Wort
25 gm. Bedstraw	30 gm. Calendula	15 gm. Dandelion roots
25 gm. Yarrow	30 gm. Greater Celandine	25 gm. Goat's Beard

1 heaped teaspoon of this herb mixture per cup of water is used. During the day at least 2 litres are sipped. It is important to use all or at least some of these herbs in their fresh state. Since in most cases of leukaemia the cause is found in the spleen, 6 sips of **Calamus root tea** have to be taken, too – 1 level teaspoon of Calamus roots is soaked overnight, warmed and strained the next morning. A sip is taken before and after each meal. 3 teaspoons (up to 3 tablespoonfuls can be given) of **Swedish Bitters** are diluted with 3 cups of herb tea and a part of it is drunk half an hour before and after each meal. **Swedish Bitters as a compress** is applied to the **region** of the **liver** and **spleen** for 4 hours and warm **Horsetail poultices** are recommended (see appropriate sections under the heading "General Information"). All acid fruit and juices, such as orange, lemon, grapefruit as well as salty and spicy food, sausages, fat meat should be avoided. Any amount of stewed apples can be eaten.

At the beginning of November 1978, a desperate couple came with their 6 year old son to see me: Peter W. from West Germany had leukaemia in its advanced stages. It had started in May 1978 with fever and pain in the legs. Because his condition did not improve, Peter was admitted to a hospital in Mannheim in July 1978. After an eleven weeks' stay he was discharged, but his condition had not improved. The first time I saw Peter, he had lost his hair, had dark shadows under his eyes, no appetite, was pale and tired and it could be clearly seen that he was very sick. After he had taken the first **Thyme bath** (see chapter on Thyme "directions") prepared by his parents according to my recommendation, he became more lively. He took a sip of the herb tea previously mentioned every quarter of an hour and although still very young, he watched the clock to be on time. He adhered to the prescribed diet. At the end of November 1978, his parents took him back to hospital for a blood test. The doctor was puzzled as his blood count was much better. During December his hair started to grow back thickly. His parents took him for a blood test again. The result: better than normal. The doctor did not know how to classify the unbelievable. In April 1979, Peter, a completely healthy boy, came with his parents to Traunstein,

Bavaria, where I gave a lecture. About 1800 people attended and the applause this boy received after I had introduced him and told his story, was thunderous. At the end of October 1979, he and his parents came to Pforzheim, Germany, to my lecture there which was attended by 2200 people. Here, too, I introduced the healthy boy. Peter, as he told me in his letter at Christmas 1979, still drinks the herb tea and from time to time his mother applies **Swedish Bitters** as a **compress** to his **spleen** and **neck** as well as **Marjoram oil** (the glands in the neck had been affected, too). On a piece of paper he drew in colour a Calendula, Stinging Nettle and Yarrow and wrote underneath **"My saviours"**! From time to time his parents still take him for a blood test, although Peter now is a healthy boy.

I find the medical check-ups extremely important! I also approve of the continued drinking of herb teas and the application of compresses. It shields a person from a relapse.

Diseases of the LIVER and CIRRHOSIS OF THE LIVER

1 cup of **Common Club Moss tea** drunk on an empty stomach half an hour before breakfast and another cup half an hour before the evening meal are helpful, as they swiftly relieve the shortness of breath accompanying cirrhosis and malignant diseases of the liver. 1 level teaspoon per cup of boiling water is used. **Swedish Bitters** as a compress should be applied for 4 hours during the day and warm **Horsetail poultices** for 2 hours mornings and afternoons while resting in bed and also overnight (see General Information "poultices" and "compresses"). Poultices and compresses have to be kept warm!

Diseases of the LUNGS

4 cups of **Yarrow tea** are sipped throughout the day, as well as 1 cup of **Horsetail tea** on an empty stomach half an hour before breakfast and another cup half an hour before the evening meal. During the day Calamus roots are chewed, the juice is swallowed with a little Yarrow tea and the residue is spat out. At the onset of pain, warm **Horsetail poultices** are applied to the chest overnight and possibly to the back, too. **Swedish Bitters as a compress** is applied for four hours during the day (see General Information "poultices" and "compresses").

Diseases of the LYMPH GLANDS

A bottle is filled with **Marjoram** and olive oil and left to stand in the sun or near the stove for 10 days. This oil as well as **Calendula ointment or St. John's Wort oil** is gently massaged into the affected glands (see chapters "St. John's Wort" and "Calendula").

Fresh **Plantain leaves** as well as **Butterbur leaves and Calendula stems and leaves** are washed and crushed to a pulp with a wooden rolling pin. The leaves should be wet when crushed to facilitate the crushing. The separate pulps are applied alternately to the affected glands. The patient will be able to tell which one is the most beneficial.

Should an operation have been performed already, **Swedish Bitters** can be applied as a compress for 4 hours besides the poultices, or the area is massaged gently with Swedish Bitters. Possibly **Horsetail poultices** can be applied mornings and afternoons while lying in bed for 2 hours. Internally at least 1½ to 2 litres of tea made from 300 gm. **Calendula**, 100 gm. **Horsetail**, 100 gm. **Yarrow** and 100 gm. **Stinging Nettle** – 1 heaped teaspoon per cup – are sipped throughout the day. The 3 tablespoons of Swedish Bitters as mentioned in the treatments for the preceding diseases should also not be forgotten.

In cases of malignant diseases of the lymph glands, **hard swellings** develop in **arms and legs**, the so called **elephantitis**. Arms and legs start to swell up, become insensate and hard and the patient feels them as pieces of wood attached to his body. In this case the previous poultices can be applied, starting from the glands and covering the swollen areas. Especially effective are the leaves of **Cow-parsnip** (Heracleum sphondylium) which grow in meadows and damp and shady places. This plant with its whitish, sometimes pinkish flowers, is taller than most other plants in the meadows and its leaves have 5 or more indentations and look like large paws. Rabbits love these leaves and so do cows, I was told. Quite a few leaves are picked, washed and while wet, crushed and applied as a poultice which, well wrapped, is left on overnight. It gives wonderful relief.

Mallow, too, cold-soaked overnight and added to the bath water gives relief. These baths help to reduce the swellings on arms and legs. Freshly pressed **Wood Sorrel juice** applied to the hard swellings is promising, too (see chapter on "Wood Sorrel").

Diseases of the OVARIES AND UTERUS

A tea is made from the following herbs: 300 gm. **Calendula** and 300 gm. **Yarrow**. 6 to 8 heaped teaspoons of herbs are needed to make 1½ to 2 litres of this tea which is sipped throughout the day. 3 tablespoons of **Swedish Bitters** are diluted with tea and apportionately drunk before and after each meal.

In addition **Yarrow sitz baths** are taken every week (see chapter on Yarrow "directions"). The water from the first sitz bath poured back over the herbs and heated again can be re-used twice so this makes 3 sitz baths a week. If tolerated, Yarrow sitz baths may be taken every day. Warm **Horsetail poultices and Swedish Bitters compresses** are applied additionally, if there is pain (see "tumour").

Here is a letter from a woman from R., West Germany, from February 1980: "I would like to write and thank you. In December 1978 I had to stay in bed for 4 months due to 2 fractured vertebrae, therefore I had ample time to study your book. In February 1979 my sister-in-law was discharged from hospital with **cancer**, considered as incurable. My brother was told that she might live for another 4 weeks, but that nothing could be done. The poor woman could not eat. A smell of decay pervaded the room in which she lay. Then she started with the herbal treatment recommended in your book. She drank 2½ litres of tea made from **Yarrow, Stinging Nettle and Calendula**; morning, noon and evening, 1 tablespoon of **Swedish Bitters** was diluted with a cup of tea. She also applied **Swedish Bitters as a compress** to her abdomen. A short time later her appetite returned and she was able to eat. The smell of decay disappeared and dark clots were discharged from the vagina; it was the cleaning process. Today she looks after the house, cooks and goes for walks. The family doctor who had received the hospital report could not remember a case like hers, but we know that these are the miracles obtained through 'God's Pharmacy'".

Diseases of the PANCREAS

The treatment is the same as for "intestines" (see page 78).

Diseases of the SKIN

If it is a matter of a still unbroken, malignant skin disorder, the orange juice of **Greater Celandine** is dabbed repeatedly on the afflicted areas during the day. For people who have no possibility to pick the stems and leaves in the wild or in the garden, I recommend a plant of Greater Celandine be kept in a flower pot. If the affliction is already an open, foul smelling, running sore, it is alternately washed or bathed with lukewarm **Horsetail tea** and cold-soaked **Mallow tea**. Then the edges of the sore are dabbed with the orange **juice of Greater Celandine** and when it has been absorbed by the skin, **Calendula ointment** is applied (see chapter on Calendula). **Plantain leaves** (Ribwort or Common Plantain) are washed, crushed and directly applied to the open sores. Should this not be immediately tolerated, the poultice is removed, the sores are washed again and the poultice re-applied. This is continued until the affected person feels the beneficial effect. **Horsetail and Mallow tea as a compress** can be applied overnight. 4 cups of tea made from equal proportions of **Calendula, Stinging Nettle, Speedwell and Yarrow** have to be drunk daily to purify the blood (1 heaped teaspoon per cup of boiling water, infused for a short time).

Sometimes it happens that after **birthmarks and hard lumps** in the skin have been surgically removed, festering, open and weeping skin eruptions develop which can be of malignant character. These are treated the same way as the open, foul smelling running sores, previously mentioned. If these sores are covering large parts of the body, **Horsetail and Mallow baths** are taken and the patient is wrapped in a sheet overnight on which freshly crushed **Plantain leaves** are spread. Malignant skin disorders which are sharply defined, scurf-like, dark patches are on the increase; these can be brushed with fresh **Bedstraw juice** several times a day (see chapter on Bedstraw "directions"). The juice poured into a small bottle is stored in the refrigerator.

A 30 year old woman had a birthmark which was surgically removed as it suddenly started to grow and was found malignant. She had to have 4 operations, because the lymph glands were affected, too. The young woman was unable to look after her family and felt desperate. **Poultices of Plantain leaves** (see "Plantain"), bathing the wounds with lukewarm **Mallow and Horsetail tea, Thyme baths** (200 gm. Thyme per bath), 1 litre of tea made from 300 gm. **Calendula**, 100 gm. each of **Yarrow and Stinging Nettle** sipped throughout the day (1 heaped teaspoon per cup of boiling water), quickly brought relief. Exactly one month later the wounds had healed — the young woman could look after her family again. God's Pharmacy works "miracles"!

Diseases of the STOMACH

In such a case **Swedish Bitters as a compress** is applied for 4 hours during the day and if possible the 4 hours should be spent out of bed, but the compress has to be kept warm. **Warm Horsetail poultices** are applied overnight. Should severe pain occur, these poultices are applied while the patient rests in bed, for 2 hours, mornings and afternoons (see General Information "poultices" and "compresses"). Additionally 1½ to 2 litres of tea made from equal proportions of fresh **Stinging Nettle and Calendula** are sipped throughout the day. In the early stages of stomach cancer, 3 to 5 drops of freshly pressed **Wood Sorrel juice** are taken in the recommended tea every hour.

A letter written in July 1979 by a returned soldier states: "After returning from a prison camp in 1947 I had **stomach cancer**. Three doctors told me it was incurable. From sheer necessity I turned to Nature's herbs and gathered **Stinging Nettle, Yarrow, Dandelion and Plantain**, from the juice of which I took a sip hourly. Already after several hours I felt better, in particular I was able to keep down the little food I still could eat. This was my salvation. Hence I seriously concern myself with herbs and have been able to observe their wonderful medicinal properties given by our Creator! Now you will understand that I feel affinity with every person who shows neighbourly love by helping people with the medicinal herbs. Do not be discouraged by negative attacks which only come from negative people. The pleasure obtained when the herbs help are worth it."

Diseases of the TESTES

Unfortunately in recent times cases have increased where besides adult males, boys and teenagers are affected. Maybe one of the causes is the wearing of tight trousers. Sometimes weeks after an operation swellings, accompanied by pain suddenly occur in another part of the body. Nevertheless the treatment has to be continued non-stop where the trouble started, at the area of the testes. The treatment is the same as for "malignant diseases of the lymph gland" (see page 81).

Diseases of the THYROID GLAND

Deep gargling alternately with **Bedstraw and Mallow tea** is recommended. Poultices from the same herbs in their fresh state are applied overnight. The herbs are washed, crushed, applied and kept warm by wrapping a piece of cloth over the poultice. The herb residue from the Bedstraw and Mallow tea is warmed slightly, mixed with **barley flour** (available at health food stores) spread on a piece of linen, applied and wrapped up. During the day **warm Horsetail poultices** (while the patient lies in bed) are applied for 2 hours and **Swedish Bitters** as a compress for 4 hours (see General Information).

Additionally 1½ to 2 litres of tea made from equal proportions of **Yarrow, Stinging Nettle and Calendula** are sipped daily (1 heaped teaspoon per cup of boiling water). 3 times a day 1 teaspoon of **Swedish Bitters** is added to ½ cup of this tea and sipped half an hour before and half an hour after each meal.

Diseases of the TONGUE

Freshly picked finely chopped **Bedstraw** is infused for a short time, 6 to 8 cups of this tea are needed and 1 heaped teaspoon of herbs per cup is used. The tea is used as a gargle (gargle as deeply as possible) and rinse throughout the day. From time to time a sip of the tea is swallowed and the rest spat out. The swelling soon subsides, the pain alleviates, sometimes after the 4th or 5th day. In most cases no radiation treatment is necessary. Through gargling and rinsing with this tea and by drinking it, the patient soon feels free from all complaints.

TUMOURS (benign and malignant tumours)

In his writtings, the Abbé Kneipp, points out that **Horsetail** arrests the growth of every tumour and slowly dissolves it. I have gained the conviction that it works. Why has such little notice been taken of Abbé Kneipp's writings? How many very sick people could have been given a chance to live and how much grief could have been avoided!

My experience shows that **warm Horsetail poultices** are the best treatment for all tumours. A good double handful of Horsetail is put into a sieve and this is placed over a pot of boiling water (a double boiler can be used). The soft, hot herbs are placed between a piece of linen and applied to the **tumour, growth, cyst, ulcer, adenoma, melanoma, papilloma, or h(a)ematoma**. In very serious cases the application of the poultice is started in the morning while the patient is still in bed and left on for 2 hours. In the afternoon it is applied again while in bed for 2 hours, and again overnight. During midday **Swedish Bitters as a compress** is applied for 4 hours. First the area is smeared with **lard or Calendula ointment**, then a piece of cotton wool, moistened with **Swedish Bitters**, and a dry piece of cotton wool on top are applied, covered with a piece of plastic and finally well wrapped with a cloth. After removal of the compress the skin has to be powdered to prevent the development of a rash.

For tumours, ulcers and growths which are external fresh **Plantain and Cow-parsnip leaves** are applied **as a poultice** (see "lymph glands"). Regularly and continously applied, these poultices can bring about an improvement on the 5th day and a result after 10 to 14 days. The freshly pressed **juice of Wood Sorrel** (the leaves are washed and still wet put in the juice extractor) rubbed on the affected area is effective.

1 cup of **Horsetail tea** is drunk half an hour before breakfast and another cup half an hour before the evening meal. 1½ to 2 litres of a tea made from 300 gm. **Calendula**, 100 gm. **Yarrow** and 100 gm. **Stinging Nettle** (well-mixed) are drunk during the day. 3 to 5 drops of **Wood Sorrel juice** are added per cup of this tea. 6 times a day, if possible, a cup of the tea is taken in intervals of one hour.

A woman from Bavaria writes: "A short time ago, I wrote to you that our neighbour, a 48 year old man, father of 4 children, had been discharged from hospital with a **head tumour and symptoms of paralysis**, very sick and desperate. One side of his face was paralysed and the eye completely closed. From the medical side he was told he would never be able to open it again. You can imagine how pleasantly surprised we were, when several days after we had used herbs according to 'God's Pharmacy', his eye opened and he was feeling much better; even his doctor was surprised."

Mr. Joachim M. wrote to the editor of a German newspaper on June 25th 1979: "To oppose the attacks of the German press against Mrs. Maria Treben and her book 'Health through God's Pharmacy', I would like to relate my child's case: Daniela, born on August 4th 1973, was very well looked after, taken to all necessary check-ups and whenever she showed the slightest symptoms of an illness we took her to the doctor and still, no doctor saw the **deadly threat** early enough, only when it was too late. At the beginning of August 1978 the trouble was recognized. Until then our child had been very lively but now, day by day, she became more listless and tired. After renewed medical consultations, when no exact diagnosis could be established, we had our daughter admitted to a children's hospital.

After days of examinations which were almost too much for the child we were told that she had an **incurable tumour** which, with today's means, could not be removed. The chances of a cure were 2 to 5% which did not completely remove all hope. Cortisone was injected and radiotherapy applied to reduce the tumour's size so that it could be removed.

At the beginning of September 1978 an operation was tried and had to be abandoned, because the child would have bled to death despite blood transfusions. The **tumour** had spread throughout the whole **abdomen, liver, gall bladder, spleen and kidneys** were affected as well as the **aorta, the leg artery** was strangled which explained why our child did not want to walk anymore. Now the child's real misery started. You can imagine how hard this was for us. For seven weeks we were at her bedside every day, in her presence smiling and joyful. This alone demanded great emotional strength. Thus we had to watch how, day by day, our child became worse. Because of the radiation therapy and the cortisone injections she hardly ate anymore. A week after the operation she developed **jaundice**. In the beginning the doctors thought it was caused by the blood transfusions.

After several more examinations lasting for hours, it was found that the **bile duct** was blocked by the tumour; another operation was recommended. To my question if the operation was really necessary, I was asked if I wanted my child to die. It would have been an attempt which the child would not have survived. As it so happened, the operating theatre was being renovated. The doctor attending the child was of the opinion that although the operation was necessary, we should wait the 10 days, until the operating theatre was again fully usable, since optimal conditions were necessary.

On my insistence we were allowed to take Daniela home for these 10 days, since nothing could be done in that time. This was the end of September 1978. In the meantime I had heard about Mrs. Maria Treben. I spoke to her on the phone and she recommended the use of the herbs as described under 'malignant tumours' in the book 'Health through God's Pharmacy'. In our misery we did not know what to do and, in our opinion, could not make things worse, only better. As we afterwards learned, Daniela was given only till Christmas to live. Mrs. Treben had said on the phone that after 5 days an improvement should be noticed. The miracle happened.

During the 5th night the child started to cry, although minutes before it had been screaming with pain. We were the happiest people. What had happened? The blood which through the blockage had not been able to flow through the veins in the legs had started to flow, causing the sensation of pins and needles. Now we were sure that the herbs were effective. Shortly before the operation was due we noticed that the **jaundice had abated** and we cancelled the date of the operation.

In the meantime the child had lost her hair. – Shortly before Christmas 1978 we took her to Augsburg for a post medical examination and the specialist there, well-known in his field, could not find a **sign of the tumour**. X-ray pictures showed only calcified patches.

It gave us great hope. All this happened within 9 weeks approximately. Our child is very well, as well as before, and through Mrs. Treben we have enjoyed her company already 6 months longer than the doctors told us.

I would like to emphasize that Mrs. Treben's help was altruistic. – All the more I am surprised that Mrs. Treben is attacked by the German press. For this reason I have related my daughter's case. To write down everything, I would have to write a book. Once again I would like to express my gratitude for Mrs. Treben's selfless help. For my family a miracle has happened."

This report sounds very promising and one has to be of the opinion that in this case **no more complications could occur**. – The tumour which had overgrown all the **vital organs**, therefore threatening Daniela's life, had disappeared but still Daniela died more than 6 months later. Unfortunately I did not learn this from her parents, but in a very cynical way from a German newspaper reporter. – How could this have happened?

Daniela's father wrote to me about six months later. – Daniela suddenly ran a fever. He also said that she had stopped taking the herbs after the good report from the examination, then "one could not force such a small child to drink the tea". – No, one cannot. But parents with wisdom can find a way to make the child drink the tea. The disease was fatal, the doctors could not help. It was the herbs from God's Pharmacy that had brought help. They surely would have continued to help. Please read the report of Peter W. under "leukaemia".

Important Hints

The **large quantity of tea** given should be adhered to in cases of **serious illness**. Although seemingly large, the patient can easily cope with the amount, if a sip is taken every 15 to 20 minutes. This way one sip has been digested before the next follows. By drinking the tea appetite returns and the digestions improves. I think highly of **Thyme baths**, even for completely exhausted, sick people, particularly if they run a fever. The patient feels the surprisingly healthy revitalization, if not improvement. People with incurable cancer sometimes suddenly suffer from **accumulation of fluid**. In this case the drinking of the mentioned herb teas is stopped and, for 5 days, 5 to 6 cups of **Horsetail tea** are sipped throughout each day. If, after the third or fourth day the fluid retention is normal, the first tea is drunk again. Should fluid accumulate again, further applications of the Horsetail treatment are undertaken. The most important rule for all these disorders and diseases is **regular medical supervision. Only a doctor can recognize the exact state of health!**

INDEX*

*The **numbers in heavy print** refer to the detailed description in "Advice for various disorders" and "Advice for malignant diseases".

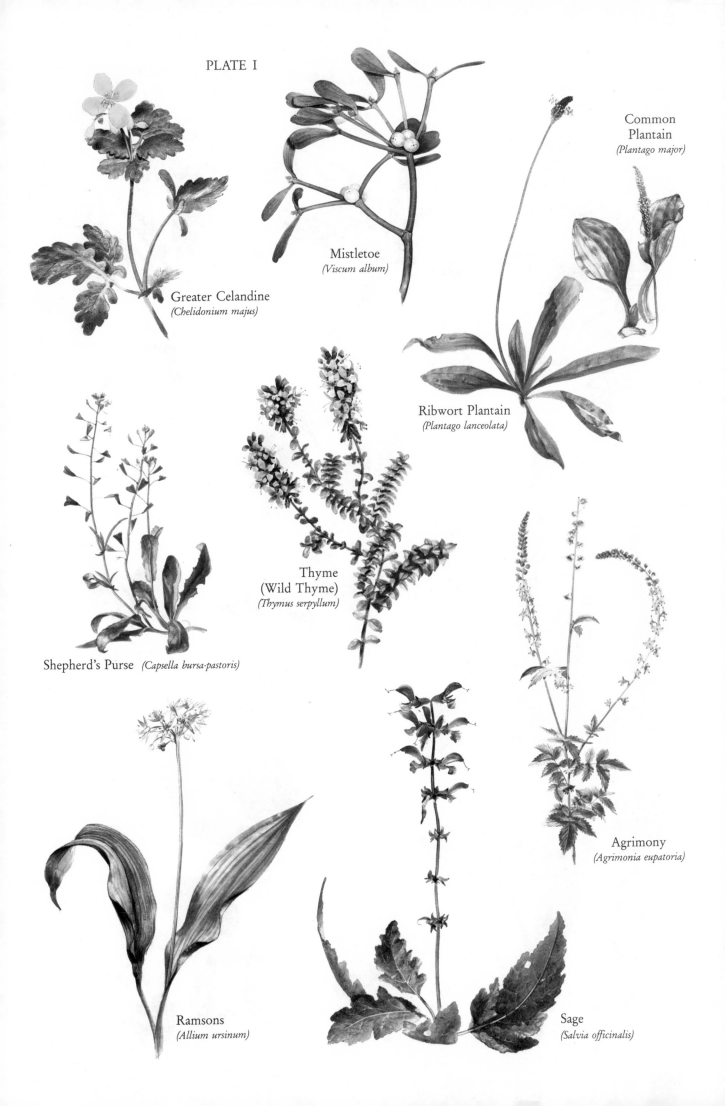

PLATE I

Greater Celandine
(Chelidonium majus)

Mistletoe
(Viscum album)

Common
Plantain
(Plantago major)

Ribwort Plantain
(Plantago lanceolata)

Thyme
(Wild Thyme)
(Thymus serpyllum)

Shepherd's Purse *(Capsella bursa-pastoris)*

Agrimony
(Agrimonia eupatoria)

Ramsons
(Allium ursinum)

Sage
(Salvia officinalis)

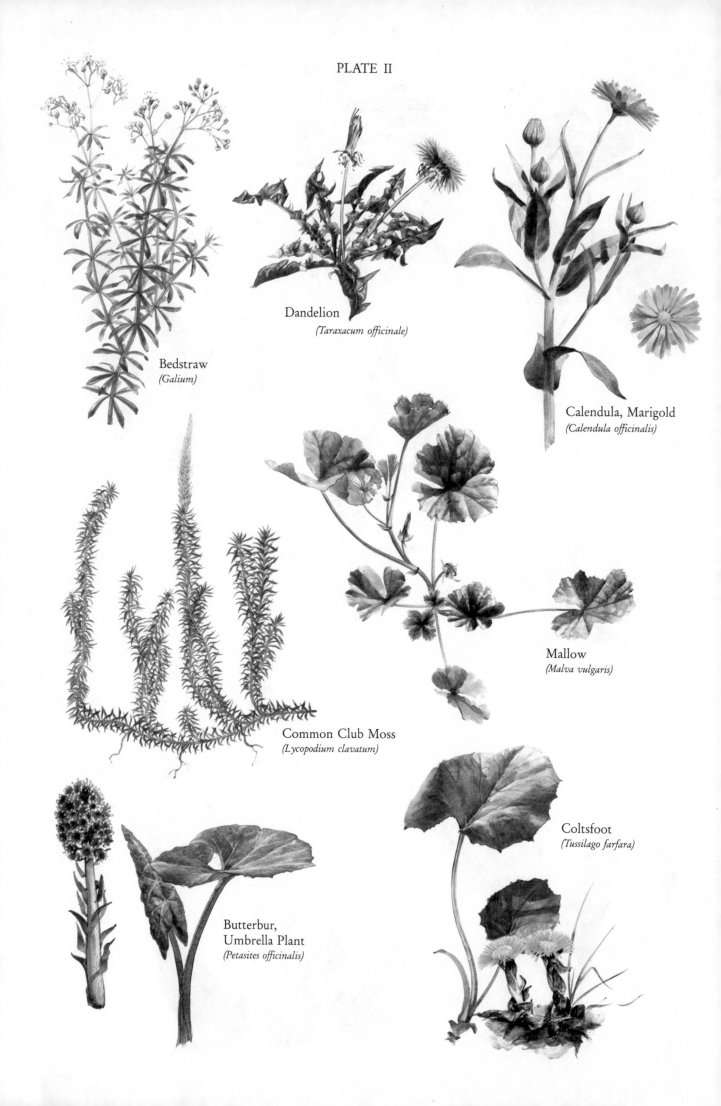

PLATE II

Bedstraw
(Galium)

Dandelion
(Taraxacum officinale)

Calendula, Marigold
(Calendula officinalis)

Mallow
(Malva vulgaris)

Common Club Moss
(Lycopodium clavatum)

Butterbur,
Umbrella Plant
(Petasites officinalis)

Coltsfoot
(Tussilago farfara)

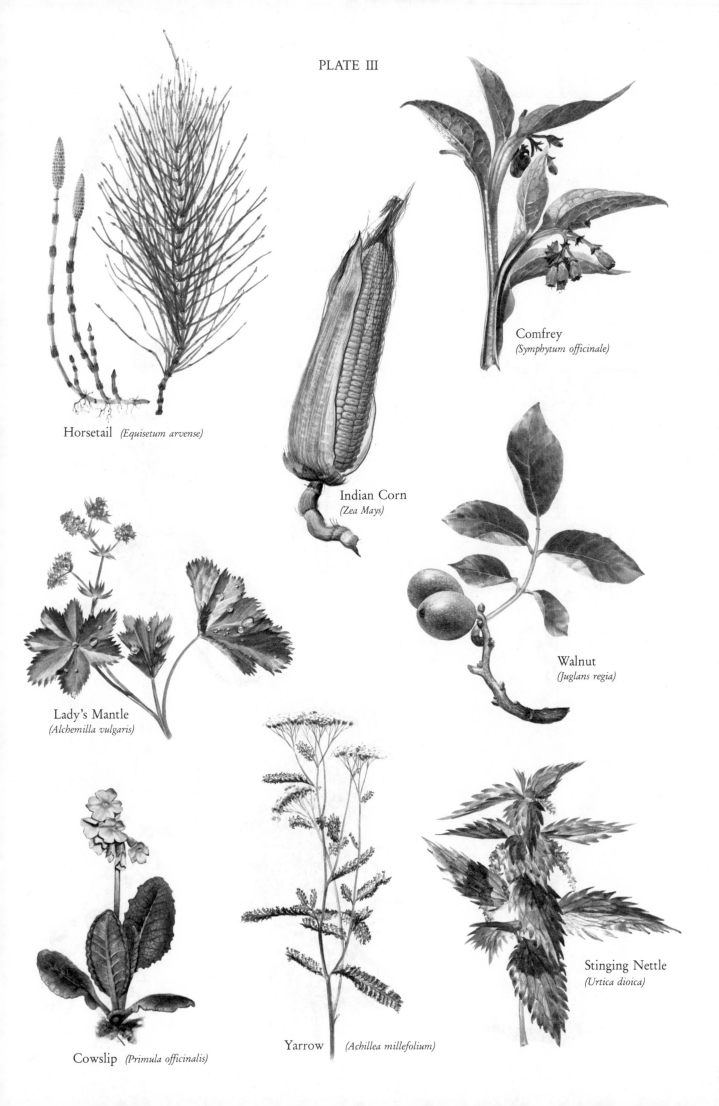

PLATE III

Horsetail *(Equisetum arvense)*

Indian Corn
(Zea Mays)

Comfrey
(Symphytum officinale)

Walnut
(Juglans regia)

Lady's Mantle
(Alchemilla vulgaris)

Cowslip *(Primula officinalis)*

Yarrow *(Achillea millefolium)*

Stinging Nettle
(Urtica dioica)

PLATE IV

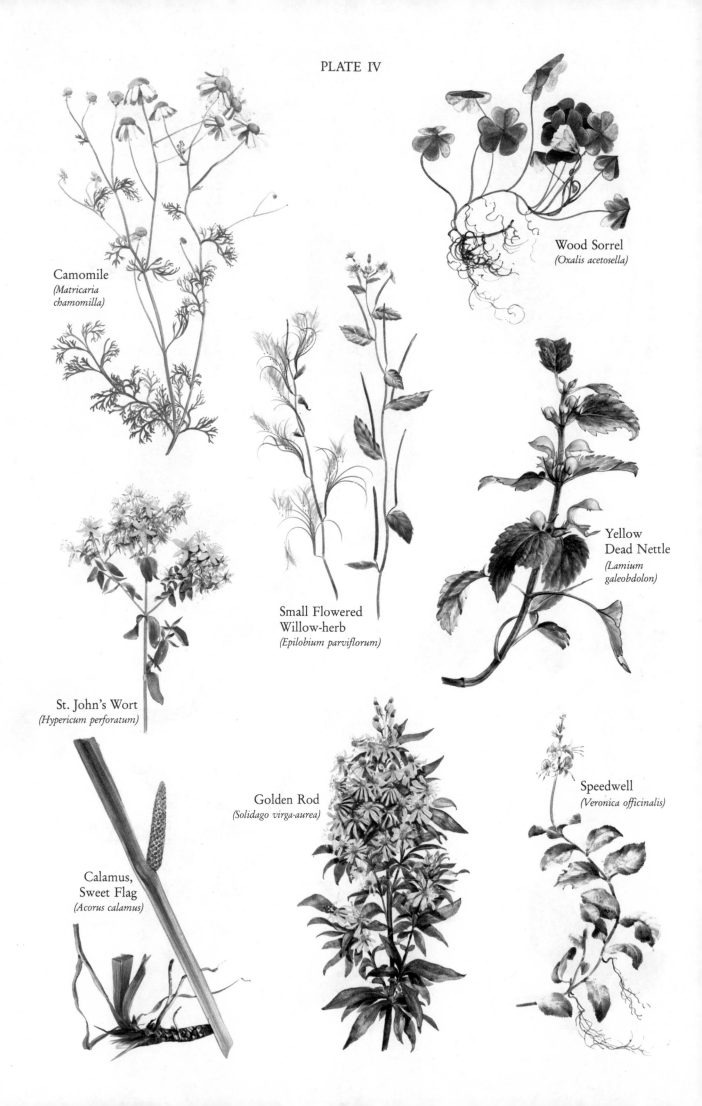

Wood Sorrel
(Oxalis acetosella)

Camomile
(Matricaria chamomilla)

Yellow
Dead Nettle
(Lamium galeobdolon)

Small Flowered
Willow-herb
(Epilobium parviflorum)

St. John's Wort
(Hypericum perforatum)

Speedwell
(Veronica officinalis)

Golden Rod
(Solidago virga-aurea)

Calamus,
Sweet Flag
(Acorus calamus)